Advancing C

Advancing Clinical Governance

Edited by

Myriam Lugon

Medical Director
Forest Healthcare Trust, Whipps Cross Hospital,
London, UK

Jonathan Secker-Walker

Senior Lecturer and Honorary Consultant
University of Wales College of Medicine,
Cardiff, UK

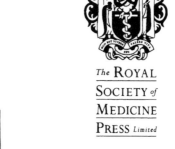

The ROYAL
SOCIETY of
MEDICINE
PRESS Limited

© 2001 Royal Society of Medicine Press Ltd
1 Wimpole Street, London W1G 0AE, UK
207 Westminster Road, Lake Forest, IL, 60045, USA
http://www.rsmpress.co.uk

British Library Cataloguing in Publication Data
A catalogue record for this book is available from the British Library

ISBN 1 85315 471 7

Phototypeset by Phoenix Photosetting, Chatham, Kent
Printed in Great Britain by Bell and Bain Ltd, Glasgow

▶ Contents

Please note: Dr Nicholas Bradley, currently listed as a contributor, co-authored chapter 10 ('Clinical Governance in Primary Care. Developing a Strategy for Primary Care Groups') with Dr Kieran Sweeney.

▶ List of Contributors

Nicholas Bradley Clinical Governance Lead, Exeter Primary Care Group, Exeter

Jane Cartwright Clinical Risk Manager, St Mary's Hospital, London

Andrew Dillon Chief Executive, National Institute for Clinical Excellence, London

Julie Glanville Information Service Manager, NHS Centre for Reviews and Dissemination, University of York, York

Dorothy Gregson Consultant in Public Health Medicine, Bedfordshire Health Authority, Luton

David Hatch Portex Professor of Paediatric Anaesthesia, Institute of Child Health, University of London, Honorary Consultant Anaesthetist, Great Ormond Street Hospital for Children NHS Trust, London

Rosemary Hittinger Imperial College of Science, Technology and Medicine, London

Susan Hobbs Chief Nurse, University Hospital of Wales, Cardiff and Vale NHS Trust, Cardiff

Sue Johnson Director, Venture Training and Consulting Ltd., Chichester

Marcia Kelson Senior Research Fellow, College of Health, London

Ann Lloyd Chief Executive, North Bristol NHS Trust, Bristol

Myriam Lugon Medical Director, Forest Healthcare Trust, Whipps Cross Hospital, London

Anna Maslin International Officer for Nursing and Midwifery, Department of Health, London

Alan Roderick Information Manager, Cardiff and Vale NHS Trust, Cardiff

Nicola Roderick Clinical Governance Analyst, University Hospital of Wales, Cardiff And Vale NHS Trust, Cardiff

Tim Scott Senior Fellow, British Association of Medical Managers, Stockport

Jonathan Secker-Walker Senior Lecturer and Honorary Consultant, University of Wales College of Medicine, Cardiff

Jenny Simpson Chief Executive, British Association of Medical Managers, Stockport

Kieran Sweeney Lecturer in General Practice and Health Services Research, Research and Development Support Unit, Royal Devon and Exeter NHS Trust, Exeter

▶ Preface

Most staff in healthcare are gradually becoming familiar with the requirements of clinical governance and what it means for them individually, for the clinical service of which they are part and the organisation to which they belong.

Over the past year, the Commission for Health Improvement (CHI) started its work of investigations and reviews of clinical governance arrangements, the National Institute for Clinical Excellence (NICE) has issued numerous Guidance to the NHS on the effectiveness and efficacy of therapeutic interventions, and a number of National Service Frameworks have been launched. This is focusing the mind of organisations that are responsible for ensuring that the services they deliver comply with and meet national standards in addition to patients' expectations. This book takes the concept of clinical governance further and addresses a number of topics pertinent to the current agenda in the NHS. As such, it covers areas not addressed in *Clinical Governance – Making it Happen*, and updates some areas covered previously. New topics covered include the nursing and midwifery contribution to clinical governance, the role of the Chief Executive, revalidation and poor performance, NICE and clinical governance in primary care. Clinical risk management – a significant component of clinical governance – is not covered directly in this book because it is discussed at length in Professor Charles Vincent's comprehensive 2nd edition of *Clinical Risk Management* (BMJ Books), published in January 2001.

This book is not meant to be a textbook and thus cover all aspects of clinical governance; it deals with issues of relevance and gives practical examples, whenever appropriate, to help the reader when taking forward clinical governance in their own organisation. It should be useful for everyone involved in healthcare, from managers to clinicians, including doctors in training who need to understand how clinical governance will influence clinical practice.

Myriam Lugon
Jonathan Secker-Walker
January 2001

▶1

Introduction

Myriam Lugon and Jonathan Secker-Walker

Change is inevitable. In a progressive country, change is constant.

Benjamin Disraeli, October 1867

Society's view of clinicians has recently undergone a sea change. This has followed from a series of high-profile medical disasters, which have received considerable media publicity. This has forced the present government and the NHS to be seen to be putting their house in order. Clinical governance became an integral part of the 1999 NHS Act. As a result, in the past two years a deluge of new guidance has been published and new institutions have been formed that have either begun to work or are about to do so. These organisations include the following:

▶ The National Institute for Clinical Excellence (NICE)

▶ Publication of National Service Frameworks (NSFs)

▶ The Commission for Health Improvement (CHI)

▶ The National Clinical Assessment Authority

▶ The NHS Plan

▶ General Medical Council plans for revalidation of doctors

▶ Corporate governance, controls assurance and standards

Whilst it may be possible to accommodate this degree of change in terms of structures and policies within a relatively short time, it is unlikely that the important change needed in culture and attitude will occur so quickly, and the government's original timetable of a decade is probably realistic.

Some significant problems need to be resolved as quickly as possible: First, time and support are needed for the extra responsibilities required of clinical directors to deliver clinical governance. Second, there is a relative lack of good clinical information to enable judgements of clinical quality to be made. Third, there is a need for easy and universal access to the Internet for clinical staff.

In most Trusts, senior doctors are faced with an increasing workload, partly as a result of political initiatives such as waiting times and waiting lists but, more importantly, because of the effect of the training requirements of junior staff and their hours of work. The days of being able to rely on a competent senior registrar to fill in whilst the clinical director is at a clinical governance review meeting are long gone. The seriousness of this problem should not be underestimated.

The amount of clinical data available and their quality are an area of concern. In the light of the recent events relating to paediatric cardiac surgery in Bristol and other enquiries relating to cardiac surgery, clinicians – surgeons in particular – are becoming less willing to take on cases with significant co-morbidity. The lack of universal codes relating to the condition of the patient on admission is an obstacle to assessing clinicians' performance in relation to the case-mix they are treating. Additionally, the degree to which a Trust's coding staff accurately reflect the written record in the secondary codes often means that the Trust with excellent coding will show up poorly compared with those Trusts who are less thorough. If patient misadventures or adverse reactions to therapeutic substances are not coded, they will not appear on the database. The amount of clinical data captured by patient administrative systems and coding at discharge can be useful for some performance indicators favoured by politicians – waiting times, for instance. However, our knowledge of outcomes is limited to whether the patient died or was discharged and to where they were discharged. There is no direct connection at present between hospital records and those in primary care, nor, as the Dr Shipman case demonstrated, any clear link between the death certification system and primary care and hospital databases.

As the numbers of externally recommended clinical standards from NICE and the NSFs grow, so the need for computer networks to make these easily available to staff becomes overwhelming. There is little doubt that the lack of networked computers and Internet access is a serious problem for many Trusts and Primary Care Groups since viewing the websites for NICE and CHI is by far the easiest method of receiving their guidance. Without the hardware and software being readily available to clinicians in their workplaces, this relatively simple method of useful clinical data capture will not be possible.

There is a common perception that the objective of clinical governance is the means by which the problem of poorly performing doctors will be resolved. Most doctors recognise that the government will continue to permit professional self-regulation on the condition that the public is satisfied that good-quality care is the norm. There is a suspicion amongst many clinical staff that the relatively few doctors practising sub-standard medicine are being used as a smokescreen to divert attention from larger problems in the NHS that will inevitably be exposed as clinical governance – and the accountability that goes with it – gathers momentum. Generally speaking, therefore, most clinical staff has willingly accepted the concept of clinical governance.

Clinical risk management, which is a significant component of clinical governance, requires untoward incidents to be reported. A common definition of an untoward incident is 'an occurrence not in keeping with the routine care of the patient or the routine operation of the institution'.[1] A 12-hour trolley wait, elective surgery cancelled on the day of operation or lack of an ICU bed fits the definition quite well. Uncomfortable as it may be for politicians of various persuasions, the past 20 years have witnessed the steady attrition of the NHS by cost improvement programmes or 'efficiency savings'.[2] These saving have been required of Trusts at a rate of about 2–3% of their budget each year. They have been presented to the public as new money being provided for the NHS and over the 20-year period will have amounted to billions of pounds. In the early years of the cost improvement programme, there was considerable spare capacity and room for improvement; however, in the past decade the cupboard has been stripped bare. Industry, passenger aircraft design, the armed services and supermarkets value the absolute necessity for spare capacity, tolerance or redundancy in order to meet the needs of the customers of the organisation most of the time. The NHS has been praised for efficiency in having occupancy rates of 97% and operating theatres and ICUs full to capacity at all times. Such lack of elasticity or tolerance in the system is actually bad for the Service and not accounted for by the supposed rise in emergency admissions or 'winter pressures'.[3,4] It is the cause of patients lying on trolleys for hours on end, then going to inappropriate wards and waiting for space in the emergency theatre. Undoubtedly, it leads to increased clinical risk to patients, poor quality care and sometimes unnecessary death.

Accountable chief executives and Trust boards are bound soon to be faced with the problem of too little resource to provide the quality of care that clinical governance demonstrates is needed. It will be interesting to see how the circle is squared.

References

1   Secker-Walker J. Clinical risk management. In: Lugon M, Secker-Walker J (eds.) *Clinical Governance: Making it Happen*. London: RSM Press, 1999: 77–91.
2   Edwards N. NHS's fundamental problems must be solved. *BMJ* 2000; 320: 1336.
3   Bagust A, Place M, Posnett JW. Dynamics of bed use in accommodating emergency admissions: stochastic simulation model. *BMJ* 1999; 319: 155–158.
4   Morgan K, Prothero D, Frankel S. The rise in emergency admissions – crisis or artefact? Temporal analysis of health services data. *BMJ* 1999; 319: 158–159.

▶2

Patient Involvement in Clinical Governance

Marcia Kelson

Introduction

Current Department of Health policy makes explicit commitments to building a health service that is responsive to the needs of patients, carers and the wider public. Key policy documents, including the White Paper *The New NHS*[1] and *A First Class Service*,[2] emphasise the importance of involving patients and the public across the range of NHS activities with the expectation that involvement should become integral to work in every part of the NHS. The most recent version of the Department of Health's Planning and Priorities Guidance[3] identifies the need to involve and respond to patients and the public as part of NHS strategies for ensuring equity of access to high-quality services. These messages are reinforced by *The NHS Plan*, published recently, which commits the NHS to 'shape its services around the needs of different groups and individuals within society. ... Patients and citizens will have a greater say in the NHS, and the provision of services will be centred on patients' needs.'[4]

A number of publications are now available which seek to provide guidance on translating the policy rhetoric on patient[a] involvement (ie patient, carer and the public) into more of a reality, by:

▶ encouraging partnerships between patients and NHS professionals[5]

▶ suggesting practical ways of involving patients in clinical audit[6] and research,[7] and

▶ advising on how best to secure patient involvement in the NHS[8] and in a range of NHS activities.[9]

Patient involvement encompasses both individual involvement (for example, the central role of patients in decisions about their own health and care) and involvement at a more collective level (patient representatives, for example, actively contributing to NHS policy and planning decisions).

Patient involvement in clinical governance

The Department of Health's framework for clinical governance and the expected benefits of involving patients in clinical governance arrangements are clearly set out in *Clinical Governance: Quality in the New NHS*:[10]

[a]The term 'patient' is used throughout this chapter to include patients, service users, carers, members of the public and members of groups representing their interests.

▶ Defined as 'A framework through which NHS organisations are accountable for continuously improving the quality of their services and safeguarding high standards of care by creating an environment in which excellence in care will flourish', clinical governance provides a means for assessing, improving and monitoring the quality of services.

▶ NHS organisations are expected to demonstrate a number of features, including 'a tradition of active working with patients, users, carers and the public'.

The document also makes explicit the benefits of change expected from involving patients:

▶ an organisation-wide strategy for involving patients, users, carers and the public, including strategic plans for communicating with them

▶ designated senior individual to oversee patient, user, carer and public involvement strategy

▶ user representatives on clinical governance committees/groups

▶ use of involvement methodologies, eg patient panels, focus groups

▶ training and education for all individuals on effective patient, user, carer and public involvement.

In attempting to involve patients in clinical governance activities in ways that are meaningful, appropriate and acceptable to both patients and professionals, NHS organisations will need to consider:

▶ why they are involving patients in clinical governance

▶ what activities patients can contribute to and when

▶ who to involve

▶ how to secure effective and appropriate patient involvement, and

▶ organisational issues, that is the extent to which the organisation is set up to support patient involvement.

Why involve patients in clinical governance?

Involving patients in clinical governance arrangements can serve different purposes. At an individual level, there is increasing agreement that involving individuals in decisions about their care increases the effectiveness of their treatment.[11] At a more collective level, patient involvement can:

▶ provide a means for NHS organisations to demonstrate accountability to the populations they serve

▶ improve staff–patient communication, understanding and relations, and

▶ engage the specific expertise that patients have to offer (for example, influencing planning, delivery and evaluation of services from the experience-based perspective of those on the receiving end of care).

Patient views on both the process and outcomes of care, and the measures used to assess process and outcomes, are needed to ensure that professionals do not make well-intentioned, but sometimes erroneous, assumptions about the quality of care delivered. Patient views are central to the definition and assessment of quality, standards and excellence – key components of clinical governance – and patients can provide their own expert views on a range of issues, including the following:

▶ Living/coping with their condition

▶ Access to services

▶ Perceived benefits and harms of treatment and care regimes

▶ Patient preferences for treatment options

▶ How well or badly treatment and care are delivered

▶ The accessibility, efficiency and effectiveness of care delivery across different sectors (eg between primary and secondary care, and between health and social services)

▶ Outcomes important to patients (including longer-term outcomes)

▶ Patient information and support needs.

Checklist 1: Why do you want to involve patients in clinical governance?

▶ To improve accountability to local patients?

▶ To improve staff–patient communication, understanding and relations?

▶ To draw on the specific expertise that patients have to offer?

▶ To improve the quality of care provided to patients

▶ To promote activities that address patient-identified needs and concerns?

▶ Other reasons?

What to involve patients in and when?

Patient experiences are considered to be a key component of clinical governance. Clinical governance involves a range of activities including clinical audit, research and development and the development and implementation of clinical guidelines. There is the potential to involve patients in all these areas:

▶ *Clinical audit:* Developments in clinical audit have emphasised the need to involve patients, as well as professionals, in all stages of the audit cycle. Patient input need not be restricted to obtaining feedback from patients, for example through patient surveys. Patients and their representatives also can be involved at more strategic levels, for example in selecting audit topics, setting criteria and standards, monitoring, disseminating findings and implementing change.[12,13] There also have been examples of patient-led audits. Salford Community Health Council, for example, has facilitated patient-led mental health service audits in adolescent psychiatry and adult forensic services.[14]

▶ *Research and development:* Historically, patients have tended to be viewed as passive participants or 'subjects' of research. Patients should, of course, always have access to full information to decide whether or not to participate in research, for example as participants in a clinical trial. However, patients and their representatives also can, if they wish, actively contribute to different stages of the research and development process itself, either as advisors to or as active members of the research team. Participation may involve contributing to identifying research topics, prioritising, commissioning, designing, managing and undertaking research, and analysing, interpreting, disseminating and evaluating research.[15]

▶ *Clinical guidelines:* Clinical guidelines are defined as 'systematically developed statements to assist practitioner and patient decisions about appropriate healthcare for specific clinical circumstances'.[16] If guidelines are to help patients, in consultation with their clinicians, to make informed decisions about their treatment and care, they need to take into account patient values and views, which are central to concepts of health, quality of life, standards of care and outcomes. Patient views can usefully inform guideline development and implementation by complementing and sometimes challenging professional views about healthcare needs.

Patient involvement does not mean that patients must be involved in every task or at every stage of clinical governance activities. However, appropriate involvement from the earliest stages will ensure that patient views inform activities from the outset. The potential usefulness of patient input at different stages is described below.

Topic selection

Involving patients in selecting topics can help ensure that NHS audit, research, and guideline and training activities address topics that patients, as well as health professionals, consider important. Patients can help prioritise areas of healthcare where they feel there is most need to improve the quality of care delivered to patients, standardise the way in which care is provided or reduce inequalities in provision.

Determining the focus and content of clinical governance activities

Patients can suggest issues and concerns that need to be addressed within the context of a selected audit, research, guideline or training topic.

Determining the measures used to set standards and assess outcomes

Patients can:

▶ identify what they consider to be acceptable and ideal levels of care to ensure that standards set address patient as well as professional measures of quality

▶ ensure that outcome measures used reflect outcomes that patients consider important, and

▶ report back on the extent to which expected standards and outcomes are achieved in practice.

Reviewing and appraising evidence

Involving patients in the review and appraisal of research evidence ensures that research findings are critiqued from a patient, as well as a professional, perspective. Both Cochrane collaboration review teams[17] and the Health Technology Assessment programme have involved patient representatives, demonstrating that they can advise on the extent to which the research evidence has addressed and taken into account patient-focused issues, including, for example:

▶ the importance patients attach to alleviating symptoms or improving health status

▶ the full range of treatment interventions and care arrangements that should be reviewed

▶ patient satisfaction with treatment and care

▶ the outcomes patients expect or desire from treatment and care

▶ the social, emotional and cultural context in which treatment and care takes place

▶ the costs, benefits and potential harms of different treatment and care options

▶ the consequences of not accepting recommended treatment or care options, and

▶ how to manage a condition where evidence of effective treatment is inconclusive or lacking.

Drawing up recommendations

Involving patients in drawing up recommendations for building on or improving the way in which care is delivered can help ensure that any changes made to services address patient experiences, needs and concerns. Patients also can report back on whether or not changes made have had the desired impact on quality.

Structure and presentation of patient information materials

The need for additional or improved patient information is often a formal byproduct of quality-monitoring activities. Involving patients in identifying their information needs can help ensure that resources are targeted on producing relevant information in appropriate, timely and patient-friendly formats.

Checklist 2: What clinical governance activities are patients involved in?

▶ Quality initiatives

▶ Clinical audit activities

▶ Guideline development/implementation

▶ 'Inhouse' research activities

▶ User-led research

▶ Training of health professionals

▶ Development of patient information materials

▶ Other activities

Who to involve?

Deciding who to involve in activities which underpin clinical governance arrangements will depend on the following:

▶ The activity or project being undertaken

▶ The input required from patients

▶ The knowledge, expertise and ability of patients to contribute

▶ The willingness of patients to participate.

There are various sources of patient input, including:

▶ Individual patients – past, current and potential patients, each perhaps having different perspectives on the delivery and provision of care;

▶ Relatives and carers – may act as proxies for patients unable to speak for themselves but also may provide information on their own expectations, healthcare needs and support needs;

▶ Advocates – ideally lay people, independent of healthcare providers or patients' families, who can relay the views of patients unable to contribute directly themselves;

▶ Patient and community organisations – range from large, relatively well-resourced national organisations with staff to small local user-led organisations. They include both condition-specific and client-specific organisations. They range from organisations run by staff or volunteers who act on behalf of a specific constituency to completely user-run and -led organisations;

▶ Community members and groups – not necessarily current recipients of services, but people from specific groups, eg people from ethnic minorities, older people, parents of young children, each of which may have views on the ways in which services, treatment and care are provided to their constituents.

Checklist 3: Who is involved in local clinical governance activities?

▶ Individual patients

▶ Relatives and carers

▶ Advocates

▶ Patient and community organisations

▶ Community members and groups

▶ Others

Note: Does the profile of patients actively involved in local clinical governance activities reflect the overall patient population profile affected by the project or initiative? If there are gaps, consider targeting underrepresented groups.

How to secure effective and appropriate patient involvement

Patient involvement in clinical governance activities can be secured at different levels:

▶ Passive input: patients provide feedback on services but have no say in what questions are asked or in how the answers are interpreted and acted on;

▶ Active participation: patients identify issues that inform the ways in which information is collected and acted upon; and

▶ Partnerships: patients work with professionals to determine the scope, focus and outcomes of an initiative.

Methods for involving patients include:

▶ patient surveys

▶ case studies, observational studies, patient tracking, patient stories and diaries

▶ workshops and conferences

▶ patient councils and panels

▶ consultation with patient representatives and groups, and

▶ recruitment of patients onto clinical governance committees and groups.

Choice of methods will depend on a number of factors, including:

▶ the purpose of the initiative

▶ the types of patients who are to participate. (Methods suitable for engaging the views of the majority of patients may not be suitable for all. Methods selected should not exclude key interest groups: additional support or alternative methodologies may need to be used to target the views of groups with special needs[18])

▶ staff expertise in different methodologies, and

▶ the preferences of patients for different methods.

Patient surveys

Patient surveys can be used to ensure that patients' views and experiences are collected to inform clinical governance activities.

▶ Quantitative surveys (eg structured questionnaire and telephone surveys) can be used to canvas the views of a relatively large number of people.

▶ Qualitative techniques (eg in-depth interviews and focus groups) involve smaller numbers of people but enable patients to explain or qualify their answers and to raise issues and concerns which NHS professionals may not have considered. Qualitative techniques also are useful to engage the views of people who may be unable to complete a structured questionnaire (eg people with poor literacy skills, non-English speakers, people with learning disabilities, and so on).

▶ A combination of techniques also can be useful. For example, qualitative methods can be used to identify issues that selective patients consider important. These can then be incorporated into a more structured survey for testing out on a larger sample of patients representative of the wider patient population.

Qualitative techniques need not be confined to obtaining patient views. They also can be used to secure more strategic input, for example by drawing up patient-centred recommendations or standards, to inform clinical governance activities. In a review of standards for professional practice, for example, the Chartered Society of Physiotherapists (CSP) commissioned the College of Health to carry out focus groups with patients to ensure that the draft standards reflected the needs of both patients and professionals. Participants in the focus groups were asked to describe their experiences of physiotherapy services, and draw on both good and bad examples of care to make recommendations to the CSP about future standards for physiotherapy services and practice.

The patient recommendations complemented similar work with clinicians so that patient and professional views jointly inform the development of the draft standards. The impact of involving patients in this exercise has been to ensure that patient perspectives on standards are addressed. Moreover, some patient recommendations have helped to strengthen the case for standards over which professionals were divided, providing a mandate for their inclusion.

Case studies, observational studies, patient tracking, patient stories and diaries

These methods can be used to see what happens to people as they engage with health services.

Observational studies tend to involve recording what happens to patients at a particular point in time (for example, recording events in a surgery, outpatients department or on a ward), whereas patient tracking usually involves recording what happens to patients at different points in their care (eg on admission, while in hospital and after discharge). While these activities are often carried out by healthcare staff, more active patient involvement – and sometimes a different perspective – can be secured if patients themselves record what happens either in the course of their own care or by observing the environment of care for other patients.

Patient stories can be collected to provide information in patients' own words about their experiences of care. Patient diaries (written or recorded onto tape) allow patients to record experiences and changes in circumstances over time.

Workshops and conferences

Patients also can be invited to participate in workshops and conferences organised to inform clinical governance activities. Inviting patients to participate in such events alongside professionals can help ensure that all stakeholders have opportunities to discuss and understand each other's viewpoints. It is important to distinguish between consultative events (where patient views are collected but patients have no opportunities to contribute to the decisions made as a result of the workshop), and collaborative events (where patient participants actively contribute to recommendations made at the conference or workshop).

The ASQUAM (Achieving Sustainable Quality in Maternity) project, for example, demonstrates how patients have participated on an equal footing with professionals in events designed to set clinical audit standards for maternity services in Stafford.

▶ Clinical audit standards were set annually by conference participants.

▶ Conference participants included representatives of all professional groups involved in providing maternity care but also members of local branches of the National Childbirth Trust, local Community Health Councils and members of national maternity and patient organisations.

▶ Participants split up into ten topic working groups, and each group sets two audit standards they would like to see adopted.

▶ All participants voted on the 20 proposed standards and the top ten were adopted for audit purposes.

Equal participation and voting rights gave patients the opportunity to influence the focus and wording of proposed standards, to suggest their own standards and to contribute to the process used to adopt the standards.

Patient councils and panels

Patient councils and panels provide opportunities for a group of people to meet at regular intervals over a period of time. Setting up a council or panel to inform clinical governance arrangements provides healthcare organisations with the opportunity to engage a formally convened group of patients on an ongoing basis (as distinct, for example, from one-off focus groups). Documented experiences of patients involved as members of patient liaison groups and councils set up by some Royal Colleges have provided some criteria for successful and effective working. There should be:[19]

▶ an explicit remit for the group with clear terms of reference

▶ clear membership criteria for all members (including professionals, if relevant)

▶ regular attendance and finite terms of office

▶ a range of interests represented appropriate to the tasks of the group

▶ established links between the group and other initiatives within the organisation

▶ mechanisms within the organisation to ensure that the groups activities are disseminated and acted upon

▶ resources, training and administrative support for the group, and

▶ monitoring of the group's effectiveness and the organisation's responsiveness to it.

Consultation with patient organisations

Patient organisations, many of which are led by users, have grown in both number and impact. Their common goals are to provide information and support to their members and to provide information to the public, raise awareness and influence professionals and policy makers.[20] Many have access to members and sometimes to paid staff who can draw on their networks to inform clinical governance initiatives directly about patient experiences of, and views on, the quality of care received. It is important to consult with as many relevant patient organisations as possible, as some will have different agendas and views to others (in the same way that some professional groupings do).

Patient membership of clinical governance committees and groups

The NHS Executive guidance on clinical governance requires all NHS organisations 'to establish clear accountability and working arrangement[s] for clinical governance' and to 'give consideration to how they can best ensure public and user input into high level discussion about the development of clinical governance'.[10] Clinical governance committees and groups should involve representatives of all key stakeholders likely to be affected by their activities, including patients. The input of patient members may be similar to that of a patient organisation (indeed, patient members may be recruited from patient organisations). However, membership of the steering group ensures that a patient perspective informs all the activities of the group, not just those discussed when the group decides to consult patient representatives on an occasional basis.

It is impossible for one or two patient members to be wholly representative of the wider patient population (in the same way that professional members of the group are unlikely to be fully representative of their constituencies). All members of the steering group, including the patient member, need to be clear about whether the patient members are there to provide a personal perspective or to draw on the views of a larger patient network. A similar case could be made for explicitly defining the role of professional members. Where patient members are asked to engage the views of a larger patient constituency, they may need resources or administrative support to enable them to consult effectively with other patients.

Checklist 4: How are patients involved in clinical governance activities?

▶ Patient surveys (quantitative and qualitative)

▶ Case studies, observational studies, patient tracking, patient stories and diaries

▶ Workshops/conferences

▶ Patient councils or panels

▶ Consultation with patient representatives and groups

▶ Recruitment of patients onto clinical governance committees and groups

Note: Consider the extent to which patients can influence the process. For example, is patient input limited to providing feedback on issues identified and acted upon by health professionals and researchers? Do patients have opportunities to influence what information is collected and how it is analysed, disseminated and acted upon?

Organisational issues

In developing an infrastructure to support patient involvement in clinical governance arrangements, there are a number of organisational issues that may need to be addressed:

▶ A clear commitment and explicit policy may help ensure that all those working within an organisation, as well as patients and patient groups who participate in clinical governance activities, are clear about the organisation's commitment to patient involvement.

▶ A dedicated budget can help ensure that resources are available to support patient involvement. The kinds of resources needed will include:

▶ the costs involved in, for example, setting up and running activities such as focus groups and workshops

▶ reimbursement of expenses of patients who participate in ongoing activities; for example, patient panel members or clinical governance committee members, and

▶ staff time and administrative costs. Organisations should not underestimate the resources needed to support the time and commitment of staff who have responsibilities for leading and engaging in patient-involvement activities.

▶ Induction, training and support also may be needed, both for staff and for involved patients.

▶ Community and user group links are also useful for ensuring that the organisation can readily consult with groups representing local patients, and patient groups can themselves approach the organisation.

Information on formal patient groups can be obtained from sources such as NHS Direct, the Health Information Service, the Council for Voluntary Services (CVS) and local libraries. However, a regularly updated inhouse database will reduce reliance on external organisations and help the organisation build up networks with informal patient and community groups.

▶ A commitment to act on patient input, together with mechanisms for reporting back to involved patients, will help to secure ongoing involvement, especially where the organisation makes an effort to evaluate patient involvement activities (with examples of improvements made as a result).

▶ User feedback on how to build on or improve patient involvement also will contribute to a developmental approach to the organisation's responsiveness to patient views.

Checklist 5: Organisational strategies for supporting patient involvement in clinical governance

▶ An explicit user-involvement strategy or policy

▶ A dedicated budget

▶ Induction, training and support (for both professionals and involved patients)

▶ Local user/community group links

▶ A commitment to act on user input

▶ Mechanisms for reporting back

▶ Inbuilt evaluation of activity (with examples of improvements made as a result)

▶ User feedback on the organisation's responsiveness to user views

Conclusion

Patient involvement should not be seen as an end in itself but as a useful tool for securing quality services for patients. This chapter has tried to provide a framework for patient involvement in clinical governance arrangements, focusing on why, whom and how to involve patients in developing quality services. Key questions facing NHS organisations involved in implementing clinical governance include the following:

▶ Do you know what patients think of services delivered by the organisation?

▶ Does the organisation engage the views of a *range* of patients, both individuals and representatives from groups representing patient interests?

▶ Does the organisation use a range of methods that are appropriate to the aims of the initiative and appropriate for engaging the views of the patients involved?

▶ Are there mechanisms in place to ensure the organisation acts on patient input?

▶ Does the organisation routinely monitor and evaluate patient-involvement activities and the impact those activities have on the quality of care delivered to patients?

In this chapter, I have attempted to provide some practical advice on how to engage patients' experiences and actively involve patients in activities that contribute to clinical governance. However, developing effective patient involvement in clinical governance arrangements will require time, effort, skills and resources. If patient involvement is to extend beyond the confines of some committed and enthusiastic NHS organisations to become a systematic and integral part of everyday NHS activity, there is a need for more evaluation of patient-involvement activities and greater dissemination of examples which produce demonstrable improvements in patient care.

References

1 Department of Health. *The New NHS. Modern. Dependable.* Command paper 3807. London: The Stationery Office, December 1997.
2 Department of Health. *A First Class Service: Quality in the New NHS.* Wetherby: Department of Health, 1998.
3 Department of Health. *Modernising Health and Social Services: National Priorities Guidance 2000/01–2002/03.* London: Department of Health, 1999. URL www.doh.gov.uk.
4 Secretary of State for Health. *The NHS Plan: a Plan for Investment, a Plan for Reform.* London: HMSO, 2000.
5 Department of Health. *Patient and Public Involvement in the New NHS.* Wetherby: Department of Health, 1999.
6 Kelson M. *Promoting Patient Involvement in Clinical Audit: Practical Guidance on Achieving Effective Involvement.* London: College of Health, 1998.
7 Standing Advisory Group on Consumer Involvement in the NHS Research and Development Programme (now Consumers in NHS research). *Research: What's in it for Consumers?* Leeds: NHS Executive, 1998.
8 Kelson M. *User Involvement: A Guide to Achieving Effective User Involvement Strategies in the NHS.* London: College of Health, 1997.
9 Barker J, Bullen M, de Ville J. *Reference Manual for Public Involvement*, 2nd edition. Bromley: Bromley Health, 1999.

10   NHS Executive. *Clinical Governance: Quality in the New NHS*. Wetherby: Department of Health, 1999.

11   NHS Executive. *The Patient Partnership Strategy*. Leeds: NHS Executive, 1996.

12   Kelson M. User involvement in clinical audit: a review of developments and issues of good practice. *Journal of Evaluation in Clinical Practice* 1996; 2: 96–109.

13   Clinical Outcomes Group. *Clinical Audit in Primary Care*. Report of the COG Primary Health Care Clinical Audit Working Group. Leeds: NHS Executive, 1994.

14   Salford Community Health Council. *The Involvement of Salford People in Health and Health Care: An Audit of Activity by Local Organisations*. Manchester: Salford CHC, 1999.

15   Hanley B, Bradburn J, Gorin S *et al*. *Involving Consumers in Research and Development in the NHS: Briefing Notes for Researchers*. Winchester: Consumers in NHS Research support Unit, 2000.

16   Field M, Lohr K. *Guidelines for Clinical Practice: from Development to Use*. Washington D.C.: National Academy Press, 1992.

17   Kelson M. Consumer collaboration, patient-defined outcomes and the preparation of Cochrane Reviews. *Health Expectations* 1999; 2: 129–135.

18   Kelson M. *A Guide to Involving Older People in Local Clinical Audit Activity*. London: College of Health, 1999.

19   Kelson M. *Consumer Involvement in the Audit Activities of the Royal Colleges and Other Professional Bodies*. London: College of Health, 1996.

20   Wilson J. Acknowledging the expertise of patients and their organisations. *BMJ* 1999; 319: 771–774.

▶3

The Organisation and Clinical Governance

Myriam Lugon and Jonathan Secker-Walker

Introduction

The duty of quality placed on Trusts is described in section 18 of the Health Act 1999:

> It is the duty of each Health Authority, Primary Care Trust and NHS Trust to put and keep in place arrangements for the purpose of monitoring and improving the quality of healthcare which it provides to individuals.

This has been a legal duty for NHS Trusts since April 1999 and is delivered through the various components of clinical governance. The Chief Executive is now accountable for ensuring that there are the systems in place that monitor the quality of clinical practice, and for assuring the Trust board that care is being delivered to patients humanely, safely and effectively, by staff who remain at the forefront of their profession. The new legislation requires the Chief Executive not only to sign the annual financial report, which guarantees probity in the handling of public money by the Trust, but also a similar guarantee in relation to the quality of clinical care.

The introduction of clinical directorates as the means of managing a complex organisation simplifies the vertical chain of command, and provides clarity as to where the responsibility for delivering clinical governance lies. However, these vertical management columns tend to make management of horizontal problems – control of infection, for instance – more difficult. There are usually several quality-related committees that focus on problems occurring horizontally across the Trust. Examples would be infection control, blood transfusion, medical records, drugs and therapeutics, radiation protection, and theatre users, and all of these committees have a valuable role to play in providing information about the quality of care. In many Trusts, when directorates replaced the cogwheel system, administrative assistance to these committees was cut to save money. In most cases, these committees did not die but had no support and no formal structure to which to report. Hence, for the last half-decade, many have functioned in a relative vacuum and often have not been as effective as they could have been.

Changes during the 1990s

The changes at the beginning of the 1990s included the introduction of clinical audit, the loss of crown immunity from prosecution for health and safety failure and the introduction of crown indemnity for NHS doctors. These all brought new quality committees into being: audit, risk management, health and safety requirements and latterly, the management of legal claims.

The clinical governance lead therefore has available a considerable quantity of existing but disconnected information about the quality of care. The framework for governance needs to provide a structure that ensures that all these quality committees make regular reports, are properly serviced and produce minutes that show clear recommendations and responsibilities for action.

The ideas explored in this chapter are personal to the authors in the light of the events of the past two years. Clinical governance is still a relatively new concept, and there is no 'right' way to manage it, although it is likely that common patterns will evolve. This chapter describes the organisational infrastructure required to deliver this agenda, the individuals/teams/organisations' responsibilities, and the place of quality in performance management.

Organisational infrastructure

The Trust board and the Chief Executive need to be confident that clinical quality is monitored and that they are provided with regular reports to warn of problems or deficiencies, in much the same way that monthly financial reports are scrutinised. It is important that the Trust board and Chief Executive decide the nature of the information that they require on a regular basis.

Monitoring of clinical quality depends on a standard against which to measure. It is often the case that Trusts have no formal mechanism for setting Trust-wide clinical policy. Individual directorates may work to guidelines – for instance, the treatment of asthma in general medicine – but often these guidelines fail to cross directorate boundaries when orthopaedic or mental health patients happen to suffer from asthma. The guidelines that are likely to be produced by the National Institute for Clinical Excellence (NICE) will need to be accepted formally (or possibly rejected if there are particular reasons), adopted and publicised by Trusts to form Trust protocols.

There is probably sense, therefore, in ensuring that the clinical governance structure recognises and encompasses two distinct components: those of *clinical policy setting* and those of *clinical policy monitoring*. The Clinical Governance Committee may undertake both these roles and ensure that the Trust board evolves a process whereby Trust policy is adopted, promulgated and monitored.

Clinical Governance Committee

This Committee should be responsible for gathering data from existing quality committees, risk management, complaints, claims and other information sources. It would be responsible for the following:

 Ensuring that the clinical performance and quality monitoring and reporting mechanisms are properly established and working.

▶ Testing the framework and process for delivering clinical governance and identify areas in need of strengthening.

▶ Receiving national guidance (eg from NICE and National Service Frameworks [NSFs]) and ensuring that they are dealt with effectively by the Trust.

▶ Developing key performance indicators to ensure the effectiveness of clinical services.

▶ Monitoring the objectives and performance of key groups and committees who are responsible for developing clinical governance across the Trust.

▶ Receiving and examining reports on the components of clinical governance, including clinical audit and clinical effectiveness, patient and consumer feedback, complaints, risk management, health and safety, benchmarking against national standards or against other similar Trusts, incident reporting, claims and litigation and continuing professional development (CPD).

▶ Ensuring that lessons are learned and practice changes are implemented.

▶ Ensuring arrangements are in place to deal effectively with poor performance.

▶ Monitoring the management of clinical competence in the Trust.

▶ Agreeing initial responses to the Commission for Health Improvement (CHI).

▶ Engaging with Health Authorities and primary care or local health groups in pursuit of the development and maintenance of appropriate frameworks for seamless clinical governance in primary, secondary and tertiary care.

Membership of the Clinical Governance Committee needs to reflect both the vertical responsibilities for the quality of care as well as those charged with horizontal issues such as the maintenance of high-quality medical records. Membership is likely to include the clinicians responsible for clinical audit, risk management and claims management and/or the clinical governance lead for the service. A university member is appropriate for teaching hospitals and the chairman of the medical staff committee or other 'unbiased' senior doctor may reassure consultant staff as to the Committee's activities. Most Trusts are likely to involve at least one non-executive director and (until their abolition) a CHC (Community Health Council) representative. The membership of the Medical Director and the Director of Nursing is crucial to the Committee.

The Clinical Governance Committee should receive the information – with recommendations from minutes where appropriate – from the following groups:

▶ Infection control

▶ Resuscitation

▶ Medical records

▶ Blood transfusion

- Drug and therapeutics
- Health and safety
- Clinic audit
- Clinical claims review
- Radiation protection
- Complaints and patient satisfaction
- Pathology users
- Theatre users.

The function of these committees needs to be made explicit and a relevant work programme agreed so that they contribute to the overall clinical governance agenda.

Some Trusts have made the Risk Management Committee responsible for receiving and prioritising the output from specialty committees in order to bring the clinical governance committee's agenda to a manageable length.

Reports that impinge on the function of the Trust should be presented to the committee such as Speciality Advisory Committee (SAC) reports on junior staff training, reports of Health and Safety Executive inspections, post-graduate deans visits and clinical pathology accreditation visits to pathology laboratories. In addition, it is likely, as a result of the publication of *An Organization with a Memory*,[1] that certain clinical incidents will be required to be reported to the Department of Health, and the Clinical Governance Committee will need to receive these reports.

An example of reporting infrastructure is shown in Figure 3.1.

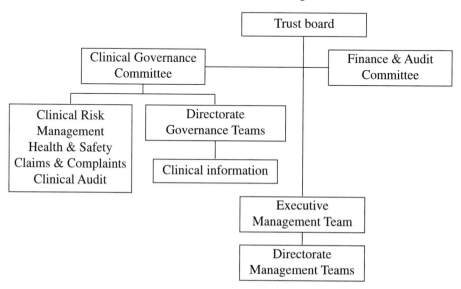

Fig. 3.1.   An example of the clinical governance reporting structure.

Delegated responsibilities

The Chief Executive is the officer accountable for the delivery of high standards of care. He/she will need to identify the clinical lead, however, to take the process forward within the organisation; this must be a board-level post. The Executive Officer with responsibility for clinical governance often is the Medical Director, but some Trusts have entrusted this to the Director of Nursing to whom, very often, many of the staff associated with quality-monitoring jobs are accountable managerially. At executive and board level, both clinical executive officers are members in any case, and both groups would expect a consensus opinion to come from these two individuals.

The lead will need to work very closely with their opposite numbers and with the Human Resources Director to ensure that clinical governance is included in an overall organisation and development plan.

The lead not only will need to ensure that the reporting arrangements are clear and satisfy the board that the appropriate processes are in place, but also investigate areas of concern and challenge clinical practice whenever necessary. The partnership between the Nursing Director and the Medical Director is critical if the delivery of this agenda is to succeed. The role of the Medical Director is described in detail in Chapter 6 and the nursing and midwifery contribution in Chapter 5.

Chief Executives should make clear to their organisations, however, that delivering high quality of care is everybody's responsibility, both at an individual and team level, and that performance management will include monitoring not only national performance indicators but also issues of clinical practice.

The Chief Executive also needs to create the right environment for clinical quality to flourish; involving clinicians in management is one way to achieve this, as is the support of a team approach to reflective learning, currently adopted by nursing. The role of the Chief Executive in this agenda is described in Chapter 4.

Role of the individual

Clinicians, in the broadest sense, are individually responsible and accountable for their clinical practice. To this end, they must ensure that they have the appropriate skills to deliver care safely and therefore ensure that their CPD programme is aimed at the maintenance or acquisition of new skills if these are required. The nursing profession has long accepted the concepts of working in teams according to clear guidelines and programmes of CPD tailored to their individual and service needs. Doctors (ie consultants) on the whole have been less formal about their practice and their personal and professional development – which has been largely left to an individual's decision.

The Trust therefore will need to establish a robust performance appraisal for all staff (including the consultants); this will help identify the needs of individuals and services as far as CPD is concerned. The annual appraisals are likely to form a major component of the proposed revalidation process. This is discussed in detail in Chapter 12.

Individual clinicians will need to monitor their own practice by taking part in clinical audit and by starting to adhere to the policies and procedures of their organisations. They also should ensure that new techniques are introduced safely and by agreement. Clinicians also will need to ensure that they fulfil the requirements for clinical supervision of junior members of staff. Many of the Royal Colleges have now produced documentation giving guidance about their expectation, such as the Royal College of Physicians on clinical governance and self-regulation[2] and the British Geriatrics Society on implementation.[3] All are available online.

Role of the clinical team

Today, care is delivered in clinical teams. Usually centred on clinical directorates and whatever the role of the board and the lead in clinical governance, the components can only be delivered by staff at the grassroots. In their document *Maintaining Good Medical Practice*,[4] published in July 1998, the General Medical Council acknowledges that care is delivered in clinical teams and that team members must demonstrate a commitment to effective clinical practice and good quality care and a willingness to learn. The Clinical Director must have access to information in order to monitor the quality of care. Much can be learnt from the analysis of incident reporting, reviewing complaints and the investigation of clinical negligence claims. However, access to clinical information also is essential. Clinical directors should be provided with the following at regular intervals:

- Patient deaths and cause of death by consultant (monthly);
- Emergency re-admissions within five days by consultant (monthly);
- Unscheduled returns to theatre by operating surgeon and consultant (monthly);
- Clinical Incidents by directorate (monthly);
- Unscheduled ITU admission from within the Trust by consultant;
- Medico-legal claims by consultant (monthly);
- Complaints by directorate (monthly);
- Data on FCEs (finished consultant episode) for top ten ICD-10 and OPCS4 codes undertaken in the directorate by consultant (six-monthly);
- Benchmarking data for directorates (six-monthly);
- Performance against publicised clinical indicators, where appropriate (six-monthly);
- Trust-wide performance against NSFs and NICE appraisals and guidelines (six-monthly).

Comparative benchmarking of data often is contracted-out to a commercial IT company. This has the disadvantage of there being significant time lapse between the episode of care and receiving the information; but there is the benefit of regular benchmarking of activity and quality measures for specialties against Trusts of a similar size and casemix. Information is discussed in more detail in Chapter 9.

At a service level, the clinical team must ensure that clinical policies agreed at an organisational level are implemented; this may require the development of care pathways or guidelines. Where appropriate, these should address the whole continuum of care from the GP practice, through the Accident and Emergency Department or the Outpatient Clinic, to the inpatient stay and back to primary care. Services therefore may need to identify how they secure the advice and support of primary care for such development, and thus address clinical governance issues across the interface. It may be appropriate for some conditions to include the steps taken in tertiary care and clarify the interface between primary, secondary and tertiary care. Addressing the whole continuum of care may require addressing social care needs for clients groups such as children and the elderly. And so on. This approach is likely to become more important as long-term service agreements based on integrated care pathways, where appropriate, become the way services are commissioned.[5]

Teams also will need to demonstrate that the care given meets the patients' needs and delivers good outcomes – although these often are difficult to quantify. To achieve this objective requires a process, at service level, to examine why untoward events, complaints and claims are occurring, to identify trends and the action required to put things right. Implementation of national guidelines and health and safety issues also should be monitored.

Services therefore should set up multidisciplinary clinical improvement groups (CIGs) or clinical governance teams (CGTs)[6] to receive their respective specialties' information on audit, risk management, claims and complaints. This group should be charged to identify any action required and any training needs, and link these to their training and education plan, to decide their audit priorities and consumer surveys requirements. An example of terms of references and composition of such a group is given in Box 3.1 and illustrated in Figure 3.2 below.

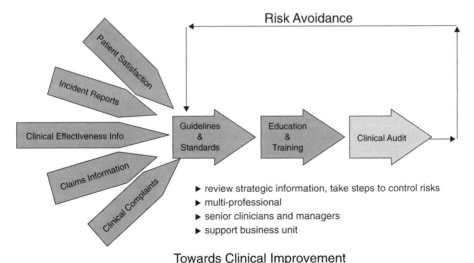

Fig. 3.2. Clinical improvement groups. Reproduced with permission from C Burke and M Lugon, © HRRI.

Box 3.1. Clinical improvement groups or directorate clinical governance teams

Membership

▶ Multidisciplinary representation including nursing, doctors, and professions allied to medicine (PAMs); it should include the risk manager, health and safety advisor, directorate manager and directorate leads on clinical risk and clinical audit.

▶ The group should be chaired by the clinical director or by the nominated directorate lead for clinical governance.

Objectives

▶ To review clinical information, identifying potential problem areas and making recommendations to the Clinical Director.

▶ To advise management on what additional clinical information is required.

▶ To coordinate clinical risk assessment in the directorate and oversee implementation of appropriate action.

▶ To ensure that all clinical areas are aware of potential risk to patients and staff.

▶ To review clinical incidents, claims and complaints in the directorate, and identify trends and remedial action to be taken.

▶ To meet the relevant standards required by the CNST (Clinical Negligence Scheme for Trusts) or Welsh Risk Pool.

▶ To review customer satisfaction surveys and identify service changes required.

▶ To make recommendation to the Clinical Director about actions to improve clinical practice and minimise risk such as development of standards/guidelines, development of care pathways, and development of appropriate clinical policies and procedures.

▶ To identify appropriate training needs required in order to change practice and ensure that they are part of the directorate-training programme.

▶ To keep written records of meetings with recommendations and responsibility for action.

▶ To ensure that minutes are kept for clinical audit meetings.

▶ To monitor the progress of annual appraisal and CPD for all staff.

▶ To ensure that clinical governance requirements are part of the directorate business plan.

Frequency of meeting: probably monthly.

The activity of the group should be open and transparent, and thus be recorded. For issues crossing more than one specialty, the chair of the committee/group (often the Clinical Director) should be given the responsibility to negotiate with other directorates. Such groups should be part of mainstream clinical business and the issues raised by quality monitoring should be addressed in the directorate's business plan. Proposed action arising should then be used on a quarterly basis for performance monitoring purpose. The lessons those groups have learnt in this process should be identified, received by the Clinical Governance Committee and disseminated to the whole organisation so that the learning can be shared and benefit everyone. Staff from clinical audit and risk departments can be developed to act as facilitators and change agents for these teams.

Role of the managers

General managers or business managers so far have found it difficult to intercede in matters of clinical practice. Whilst it is not for them to dictate how patients are treated, clearly they have a role not only within the effectiveness field,[7] but also within the overall clinical governance agenda.[8,9] Indeed, as chief executives now have statutory responsibility for the quality of care delivered, so too will managers need to understand their own responsibilities in ensuring that clinical practice is safe and adheres to the relevant guidelines. Where shortfalls are identified they will need to support the team in taking the appropriate action. Managers therefore must foster a multidisciplinary approach to patients' care; an inquisitive culture where learning and reflecting on the team and the individual's practice is part of the norm. They will need to ensure that the team adheres to the yearly individual performance review process necessary to identify training and education requirements and aggregate the individual plans at a team level to prepare a comprehensive and all-inclusive training plan. To fulfil their role effectively, managers will need to understand how clinicians function, how best practice is identified, how practice can be monitored effectively, what clinical risk management means, how complaints can be used to influence changes in clinical practice, and their own role within individual performance review. This highlights the need for managers to receive the appropriate training and development to secure understanding of these processes.[10]

A partnership between clinicians and managers is necessary for the successful delivery of the quality agenda. Managers will need to facilitate and adopt a supportive approach, but also may need to challenge clinicians constructively. This identifies the significant cultural and organisational change required[11] and must be considered by the Chief Executive and the Human Resources Director as part of the trust organisational development agenda.

Role of the organisation

While the clinical agenda can succeed only if owned by all staff, the organisation has the responsibility to ensure that clinical governance is taken forward cohesively and consistently across all services. It therefore needs to give the services and their CIGs/CGTs clear direction and goals. The organisation will need to ensure a common approach is taken, whilst allowing clinical teams to progress at a pace they can sustain, by developing a framework which shares the vision of what the organisation is aiming to achieve with regard to clinical governance. It should identify key clinical governance objectives that are the same for all levels of the organization. It should develop a structured system to measure progress in order to facilitate planning and monitoring over time. Clinical teams are then better placed to develop an action plan with leads and time scales that will guide their activities.

A framework has been proposed for supporting clinical governance in primary care, which is about establishing the baseline, putting a plan into place, acting on it using tools such as education and training, and monitoring patient satisfaction, clinical outcomes and staff satisfaction.[12] Frameworks, however, must address all the key elements of clinical governance. An example is given below, which has been developed to focus on the following: thinking on the key components and tasks of clinical governance; to allow the identification of where each service is now and what needs to be done to achieve the aims and objectives set by the organisation; to facilitate the comparison of progress made by individual services or directorates and to identify and share lessons learnt from the process. Using this framework, clinical services can develop short- to medium-term objectives for individuals, teams and directorates, which will contribute to the implementation of systems of clinical governance.

Four objectives were identified which underpin the development of clinical governance:

- Identifying and managing exceptions;
- Providing clinically effective services;
- Developing and empowering staff;
- Providing open management.

Seven broad key result areas, as shown in the box below, underpin these objectives.

Box 3.2. Clinical governance framework	
Clinical governance objectives	Key result areas
Identifying and managing exceptions	Clinical risk management
	Complaints management
Providing clinically effective services	Effective clinical audit
	Evidence-based practice fully supported
	Implementation of NSFs
Developing and empowering staff	Workforce planning and CPD
Providing open management	Professional and Trust performance procedures

The key results areas contain the indicators by which progress will be measured and are the 'technical aspects' of clinical governance. In clinical risk management, for example, one would look for the following actions:

▶ Development and application of a specialty specific procedure identifying trigger events which are then regularly reported and reviewed;

▶ Regular trends analysis of incidents leading to changes in clinical practice and/or training;

▶ Identification of serious clinical incidents and thorough investigation in accordance with the organisation's procedure;

▶ Regular risk assessment and action taken as a result;

▶ Clinical risk management included in the local induction programme and training in risk management available to all staff incidents.

The action plan for the implementation of each subsection can be developed and agreed with each directorate/service or teams, and specifies the key tasks, systems and processes that are to be established during a specific time period. It gives the clinical team the flexibility to tackle their highest priority first while ensuring that all services will, over time, have implemented the relevant systems. It also recognises that services will be at different stages of development; each plan is thus customised to individual service development needs. But the organisation can make a number of corporate tasks and time scales mandatory such as accurate recording of complications from surgical interventions and their regular monitoring and/or ensuring that lessons learnt by the activity is shared with all the staff in the directorate/service.

The CIGs or CGTs should be asked to report regularly on progress to the Clinical Governance Committee identifying the activities undertaken, the changes made and the lessons learnt, which can then be disseminated to other services, thus avoiding individual teams to duplicate effort. These groups also need to identify issues to be addressed at corporate level such as policy development, development of specific training programme, etc. Quality and clinical governance must become part of routine practice and as such should be an integral part of the business planning process and be a regular feature discussed at board meetings.

Role of the board

Non-executive directors have an important role to play in monitoring the quality of care provided by the various clinical services and in challenging individual services. To do this successfully, they must have an understanding of the processes used for monitoring, such as clinical audit, clinical risk management, and so on. Some training in these processes should probably be part of the development programme for non-executive directors, if they are to discharge their responsibility successfully. Non-executive directors should be active participants of a Clinical Governance Committee and could be used as one of the drivers to ensure successful implementation of necessary changes in clinical practice. In many cases, they may chair such a committee. It is important that they feel able to challenge clinicians and managers in a constructive and non-threatening manner and support the executive directors in their endeavour to identify warning signs of poor clinical performance, as described later on in this chapter.

Monitoring performance

Quality reporting and monitoring should become a significant part of performance review. Many of the elements determining quality can be captured from clinical risk reporting, analysis of claims and the content of complaints. (A template for quality reporting is described in Box 3.3.) For most of these elements, a trend analysis is

---

Box 3.3.   A template for quality reporting

Specialist surgery

Clinical claims

Business unit/ specialty	Total cost	Trust cost	New claims during Q2	Claims settled during Q2	Total number of claims
Orthopaedics					
Ophthalmology					
ENT					
Total					

Clinical incidents/near misses

Business unit/ Specialty	Severity						
	Death	Severe	Moderate	Minor	Near miss	Not recorded	Totals
Orthopaedics							
Ophthalmology							
ENT							
Total							

Orthopaedic incidents

Event type	Q4 97/98	Q1 98/99	Q2 98/99
Lack of team member			
Medication errors			
Equipment failure			
Other			

contd.

Clinical complaints

Business unit/ specialty	Clinical complaints code (see below)							Total
	1	2	3	4	5	6	7	
Orthopaedics								
Ophthalmology								
ENT								
Total								

Code	Description
CC1	Clinician failed to diagnose correctly
CC2	Clinician failed to treat appropriately (no treatment or wrong treatment)
CC3	Clinician performed activities outside their competence/failed to seek guidance
CC4	Clinician did not communicate adequately with patient/representative/guardian/ other clinical staff
CC5	Clinician gave incorrect information to patient/representative/guardian
CC6	Clinician had an abusive or dismissive attitude which upset the patient or failed to take into account patient or representative's sensitivities
CC7	Other complaint of a clinical nature not covered by codes CC1–CC6

Clinical complaints

Business unit/specialty	Q4 97/98	Q1 98/99	Q2 98/99
Orthopaedics			
Ophthalmology			
Oral Surgery			

Comments

necessary to determine whether the problem is one-off or recurring; the latter may warrant investigation and remedial action. A quarterly report thus is most likely to be of use. This report should form part of the performance review of the various clinical services/specialties; and whenever necessary, remedial action needs to be taken, the responsible individual and time scale for implementation needs to be identified and the actions subsequently monitored. The manager of the service should be held accountable for the delivery of the action plan.

Box 3.4. Example of audit questions

Clinical Governance Surgery

Q1 Directorate

Q2 Specialty

Director completing this form   Date: ....

This form should be completed fully and returned to the Risk Manager no later than .... (date).

Q3 Does the Service have individuals responsible for the management of the following:

	Yes	No
Clinical Risk Management	☐	☐
Clinical Audit	☐	☐
Complaints	☐	☐
Workforce planning	☐	☐
Co-ordination of clinical effectiveness information	☐	☐
Setting Service quality standards	☐	☐

Q4 Does the Service use the Trust Incident Reporting mechanism to ensure adverse events are identified?

Yes ☐
Sometimes ☐
Rarely ☐
No ☐

Q5 Are adverse events openly investigated, lessons learnt and changes made?

Yes ☐
Sometimes ☐
Rarely ☐
No ☐

Q6 Does the Service routinely assess clinical risks and put action plans in place to reduce risk to patients?

Yes ☐
No ☐

Q7 Is the quality of clinical record keeping (medical, nursing and other) routinely monitored?

Yes ☐
Sometimes ☐
Rarely ☐
No ☐

Q8 Does the Service have a clinical audit programme?

Yes ☐
No ☐

Q9 If yes, does the programme involve all relevant clinical staff (medical, nursing, others)?

Yes ☐
No ☐

contd.

Q10 Do the results of audits bring about changes/improvements to working practices?
   Yes ☐
   Sometimes ☐
   Rarely ☐
   No ☐

Q11 Does the Service routinely hold a meeting to discuss quality issues, i.e. adverse incidents, complaints, clinical audit results, etc?
   Yes ☐
   No ☐

Q12 If yes, what is the name of this meeting?

Q13 Is this meeting multidisciplinary, involving all parties including managers?
   Yes ☐
   No ☐

Q14 Does this meeting recommend changes in how services are provided and ensure these happen?
   Yes ☐
   Sometimes ☐
   Rarely ☐
   No ☐

Q15 Are you discussing quality issues as part of the Service's business planning process?
   Yes ☐
   No ☐

Q16 Below are a number of statements, please rate how strongly you agree with each statement using the scale 1 to 5, where 1 = agree strongly, 5 = disagree strongly.

	1	2	3	4	5
Evidence-based practice is supported and applied routinely in everyday practice.	☐	☐	☐	☐	☐
Workforce planning and development is fully integrated within the Service.	☐	☐	☐	☐	☐
Development programmes aimed at meeting the needs of individual health professionals and the Service needs are in place and supported locally.	☐	☐	☐	☐	☐
Processes for assuring the quality of clinical care are in place in the Service.	☐	☐	☐	☐	☐
Lessons are learnt from complaints and recurrence of similar problems avoided.	☐	☐	☐	☐	☐
Professional performance procedures that help an individual improve their performance are in place and understood by all staff.	☐	☐	☐	☐	☐
Clear procedures exist that allow staff to report concerns about a colleague's professional conduct and performance.	☐	☐	☐	☐	☐

It also will be necessary to include in the performance review process the national clinical indicators, performance framework and other measures of quality that Trusts will be asked to report to the NHS Executive. It must be recognised, however, that systems and processes to monitor quality are unlikely to be at the same stage of development across all services in an organisation. It is necessary, therefore, to audit in the first instance the baseline for services in order to identify how much help and support they need from central function in order to progress. This audit should be simple and should test not only the stage of development of each service with regard to the quality agenda but also test understanding of their responsibilities. An example of audit questions is given in Box 3.4.

Monitoring development and progress in large and complex organisations is not a small undertaking. The authors therefore suggest that a system for self-assessment for clinical governance is developed based on the UK/European model for business excellence[13] (illustrated in Figure 3.3). Processes such as clinical audit, clinical risk management, complaints handling, etc., are the enablers necessary to produce better outcomes for the patient, which is one of the key results. This approach would have the benefits of involving staff in the process of continuous clinical improvements as well as empower and motivate them. Performance monitoring requires accurate and reliable data from quality indicators that are easily and repeatedly measurable.[14] There is much to be said for amalgamating staff in risk and claims management with complaints, audit, specialised IT and quality staff into central 'governance departments' and gradually developing generic governance workers related to and very familiar with each clinical department or group.

The UK/European model

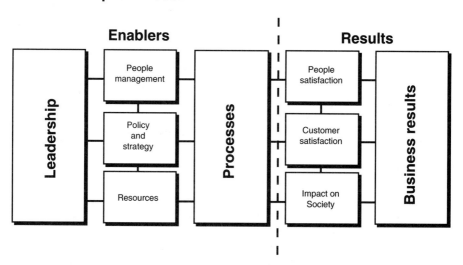

Fig. 3.3. The UK/European model. © British Quality Foundation and European Foundation for Quality Management.

Dealing with poor clinical performance

Whilst it is recognised that the majority of staff working in the NHS strive to do their best for their patients, there are occasions – as the Bristol case and the GMC cases of two gynaecologists has demonstrated – where the performance of doctors and other clinical staff is deficient. The Chief Medical Officer, in his document *Maintaining Medical Excellence*,[15] requires that healthcare organisations put in place procedures to identify and deal with performance issues early to prevent harm to patients. The British Association for Medical Managers translated this document into a procedure, which was disseminated to all medical directors. The authors suggest that this procedure be put in place in all Trusts.

The pathways for dealing with poor performance must be clear, explicit and widely disseminated and understood. As care is increasingly organised in clinical directorates, the authors suggest that the job description of clinical directors includes responsibility for dealing with poor performance and identifying remedial action. The emphasis, however, should be on prevention with identification of potential problems early. Indeed, in many recent publicised cases the warning signs were present early but seemingly were not picked up. An executive clinical governance group could fulfil such a function. The membership should include the Chief Executive, the Medical and Nursing Directors, a non-executive director on the Clinical Governance Committee and the manager heading clinical governance. This committee's role should be to identify early warning signs of perceived 'poor performance' which warrants further investigations. It should use available information such as complaints (issues within), clinical incidents and near misses, claims, mortality rate, re-admission rate and benchmarking risk management information if available by individual clinicians and teams and identify if this information considered together, suggests areas of concern for further investigation by the relevant director. Indeed the paper *Quality in the NHS: A First Class Service*[16] lists complaints, incident reporting, etc., as a way to monitor clinical performance and identify poorly performing staff. While the Chief Executive must be satisfied that clinical practice in his/her organisation is safe and of high quality, the clinical team also should consider such information regularly to ensure that lessons are learnt and training provided where appropriate to avoid repeated untoward events and damage to patients.

It is important that organisations are supportive of staff and invest in their training to avoid individuals operating at a level where they are no longer competent. However, if a serious shortfall in performance is identified through audit or clinical risk management, the individual clinician must be asked to stop the given intervention until he or she has received further training. The BMA's Central Consultants and Specialists Advisory Committee[17] has recommended that medical directors set up a professional advisory panel to investigate a problem with medical staff at an early stage. It suggests that the Chairman of the Medical Staff Committee chairs it, with the Clinical Director of the doctor concerned and a consultant from a neighbouring trust in the relevant specialty. The 'three wise men' procedure may run in parallel where physical or mental health is thought to be involved. Serious clinical incidents must be investigated looking not only at individual practice but also at organisational systems. The organisation's approach should be supportive, however, and it should be ready to deal with problem doctors or nurses before patients are damaged but should ensure that the GMC's guidance is followed. In certain circumstances, however, the procedures suggested in *Supporting Doctors, Protecting Patients*[18] will need to be invoked.

Controls assurance

Organisations need to pay attention to the relationship between clinical governance and controls assurance. Put simply, controls assurance requires the directors of Trust boards to satisfy themselves that systems are in place to ensure that all types of risks are assessed and properly managed. Initially, the emphasis is on organisational and financial controls with such things as standing financial instruction, organisational development plans and purchasing strategies being regularly reviewed and updated. In due course, this expands into other areas such as clinical risk and health and safety requirements. This is discussed in detail in Chapter 13.

Reporting to the board

As mentioned earlier in this chapter, the board will need to consider quality and clinical indicators on a regular basis; some information will be required monthly, some quarterly. It is important that the Chief Executive and the Trust Board agree the level of detail required and the type of information provided. Information and data quality is dealt with in Chapter 9. It also must be recognised that information regarding clinical incidents, claims and complaints will by definition deal with confidential data. Whilst it is accepted that the NHS must be more open, putting some of this information into the public domain could damage patients' confidence and be threatening for staff. The format for the report therefore will need to be considered carefully. In any case, the implementation of recommendations arising out of the investigations into a serious clinical incident and/or independent reviews of complaints must be monitored. The Clinical Governance Committee certainly will need to taken part in such monitoring. Reports submitted to committees and to the Trust board must not breach the duty of confidentially and should ensure that they comply with the Caldicott principles.[19] For example, a format anonymising the data, as in an Audit Commission report, could be a way forward; a fictitious example is given in Table 3.1. It will also be necessary for each Trust to develop good relationships with the local press, highlighting the need to be supportive of the organisation's approach to quality.

Whilst the information used for monitoring purposes should not identify an individual clinician, the Board may want to adopt and/or develop clinical indicators by which services can be benchmarked against nationally available information. However, it must be recognised that the use of clinical indicators to monitor quality in healthcare may not be straightforward. This has recently been discussed by Sheldon.[20] The implementation of the National Framework for Assessing Performance[21] also will lead to the production of comparative information. The board also will need to ensure

Table 3.1. Reporting and monitoring recommendations for serious clinical incidents – fictitious example

Case No.	Risk	Recommendations/control	Lead	Date	Completion
SCR 001.1	Misdiagnosis of acute pancreatitis and inappropriate management in A&E	Include diagnosis and treatment in compulsory teaching sessions of A&E SHOs	A&E consultant	Oct. 99	
		Make all SHOs in A&E aware of the investigation results	A&E consultant	Aug. 99	Aug. 99
SCR 001.2	Traumatic effects of incidents on those involved	Support individual doctor professionally and emotionally	Consultant and senior nurse	Aug. 99	Aug. 99
SCR 002.1	Risk of cross infection in theatres during eye surgery	Review of aseptic practice within theatres	Control of infection nurse	Sept. 99	Sept. 99
		Implementation of recommendations from review	Manager and consultant surgeon	Nov. 99	
SCR 002.2	Availability of specialist opinion out of hours	Circulate briefing note to all junior staff with contact out of hours for ophthalmology opinion	Clinical Director ophthalmology	Sept. 99	Sept. 99
SCR 002.3	Misdiagnosis of serious eye infection	Include in training session for SHO in ophthalmology and A&E	Clinical Director ophthalmology	Oct. 99	
SCR 002.4	Availability of medical records out of hours	Improve process for accessing medical notes	Patient's service manager	Nov. 99	

that they test services against the performance measures developed as part of NSFs. It will be important to make explicit the quality standards that can be attained given the level of resources available locally.

Conclusion

Developing and implementing systems and processes to monitor clinical performance and the quality of clinical care needs time, effort skills and resources. Much will depend on ease of access to good clinical information; an aspect of the NHS which in many Trusts is still woefully deficient. It is important that organisations recognise that clinical teams must be empowered to identify problems and deal with them but also to be prepared to celebrate successes. The development of effective clinical team working is a necessary ingredient to the successful implementation of clinical governance as well as good change management processes. Clinical audit and risk staff and those within complaints departments will need to work together closely, providing their expertise to the clinical directorates. This will facilitate changes in clinical and operational practice and help directorates deliver improved quality of care. This highlights a significant organisation and development agenda for any healthcare organisation. A clinical governance implementation plan therefore must be seen as part of an overall organisational development plan and figure in the business plan of individual services and of the whole organisation. To progress this agenda successfully, the executive team will need to pull their effort to support this process, work in partnership with clinical teams and other organisations, and recognise that its success will depend on a steady evolution, not a revolution.

References

1   Department of Health. *An Organisation with a Memory*. Report of an Expert Group on Learning from Adverse Events in the NHS. London: The Stationery Office, 2000.
2   Maintaining good medical practice: Clinical governance and self-regulation for physicians. *J R Coll Physicians London* 1999; 33(3): 241–245. URL: http://www.rcplondon.ac.uk/news/news_clin_gov.htm.
3   Guidelines for the Implementation of Clinical Governance in Geriatric Medicine. British Geriatrics Society. URL: http://www.bgs.org.uk/ 9implemr.htm.
4   *Maintaining Good Medical Practice*. London: General Medical Council, July 1998.
5   HSC 98/198. *Commissioning in the New NHS. Commissioning Services 1999–2000*. London: Department of Health, 1998.
6   Burke C, Lugon M. Integrating clinical risk and audit – moving towards clinical governance. *The Health Risk Resource* 1998; 2(1): 16–18.
7   Dunning M, Lugon M, McDonald J. Clinical effectiveness. Is it a management issue? *BMJ* 1998; 316: 243–244.
8   Ayers P. Clinical governance setting the scene. Comments. *Hospital Medicine* 1999; 60(7): 470–471.
9   Sutherland K, Dawson S. Power and quality improvement in the new NHS: the role of doctors and managers. *Quality in Health Care* 1998; 7(suppl): 16–23.
10 Heard S. Educating towards clinical governance. *Hospital Medicine* 1998; 59: 728–729.
11 Donaldson LJ, Muir-Gray JA. Clinical governance: a quality duty for health organisations. *Quality in Health Care* 1998; 7(suppl): 37–44.
12 PCG Resource Unit. *Clinical governance. Supporting clinical governance in primary care: a practical framework*. http://strauss.his.ox.ac.uk/ pcgu/clinical_governance_framework.htm.
13 British Quality Foundation (BFQ) and European Foundation for Quality Management (EFQM). *UK/European Model for Business Excellence*, 1990–1991.
14 Nelson EC, Spaine ME, Batalden PB, Plume SK. Building measurement and data collection into medical practice. *Annals of Internal Medicine* 1998; 128: 459–466.
15 Chief Medical Officer. *Maintaining Medical Excellence*. London: The Stationery Office, 1995.
16 The Department of Health. *Quality in the NHS. A First Class Service*, 1998.
17 Consultants issue guidance on professional advisory panels. *BMJ* 1998; 317: 1663.
18 Department of Health. *Supporting Doctors. Protecting Patients*. London: The Stationery Office, 1999.
19 The Caldicott Committee. *Report on the Review of Patient-Identifiable Information*. London: Department of Health, 1997.
20 Sheldon T. Promoting health care quality: what role performance indicators? *Quality in Health Care* 1998; 7(suppl): 45–50.
21 The Department of Health. *The New NHS. Modern. Dependable. A National Framework for Assessing Performance*. London: The Stationery Office, 1998.

▶4

Role of the Chief Executive in Clinical Governance: Some Practical Guidelines

Ann Lloyd

Introduction

The publication of *The New NHS. Modern. Dependable*[1] has heralded the beginning of a new era for the NHS. The Government's aim is to build a modern and dependable health service, providing a fast, responsive, high-quality service which is consistent and equitable in all parts of the country. A substantial programme of modernisation is being introduced to:

▶ improve people's health – and that of the poorest in society, in particular – by tackling the causes of ill health nationally and locally;

▶ make services quick and convenient for people to use;

▶ improve the consistency of services so that people can be sure of a high-quality service whenever and wherever they use the NHS;

▶ break down the barriers between different parts of the health and social care system so that people's needs are dealt with as a whole and without being passed from pillar to post; and

▶ modernise the NHS by investing in staff, buildings, equipment and information systems.

At the heart of these reforms is the strategy that requires the quality of care delivered to become the driving force for the development of health services. Clinical governance has become the lynch pin for that strategy.

The responsibility and accountability for the overall quality of clinical care has been placed on the shoulders of the Chief Executive of the employing organisations. This has come as no surprise to the majority of the Chief Executives in the country who always assumed that accountability. Certainly, in their experience of managing complaints and concerns from patients, they have always believed themselves to be held to account by the public for that responsibility.

Additionally, the responsibility for Chief Executives has been spelled out clearly for many years in their job descriptions, which demand that 'the role and responsibility for Chief Executives is:

▶ to provide direction, strategic vision and leadership to the organisation

▶ to manage organisational performance

to establish and maintain constructive external partnerships and collaboratives

to be accountable for the governance of the organisation.'

The really tangible change for Chief Executives arising from the publication of HSC 1999/065, *Clinical Governance: Quality in the New NHS*,[2] is that now they have to demonstrate clearly that they have mechanisms in place through which they can account for this responsibility and take action on the outcome of these processes in the organisation.

The key policy principles underpinning the elements of the strategy for developing and improving quality in the NHS are described elsewhere in this book. However, the key task for the Chief Executive in any organisation remains the creation and management of the culture through which services are delivered, and clinical governance and its management is critical to the development of that culture.

The Command Paper[1] demands that 'the new NHS will have quality at its heart. Without this there is unfairness. Every patient who is treated in the NHS wants to know that they can rely on receiving high quality care when they need it. Every part of the NHS and everyone who works in it should take responsibility for working to improve quality' (paragraph 3.2, *The New NHS. Modern. Dependable*).

It is the environment through which this strategy can be delivered that has to be developed by the Chief Executives of the organisation, in conjunction with their clinical and managerial teams.

Appropriately, the drive to implementing and maintaining improvements made in the quality and equality of the service delivered will be set within a national context. This will make clear the minimum standards expected from services, on the basis of good information and evidence, within a national overarching performance framework for monitoring the delivery of those standards.

The area with which NHS Trusts and other NHS accountable bodies have to grapple is known as 'the middle core'. This comprises the institution of mechanisms for ensuring local delivery of high-quality clinical services, through clinical governance reinforced by this new statutory duty of quality; supported by programmes of life-long learning, the local delivery of professional self-regulation and the involvement of users and their carers in the mode of delivery of the services.

The local focus – necessary action

Patients want their doctors to be well trained, up to date and professionally competent as well as kind, considerate and respectful of their views and wishes when treating them. When we are ill, we all want doctors we can trust.

The narrow view – that the medical regulation is the sole responsibility of central institution like the Royal Colleges of Medicine at the General Medical Council – misses the essential point. Doctors and other professionals and managers all have the responsibility to work together to assure and demonstrate good practice and act promptly and decisively when things seem to be going wrong.

Sir Donald Irvine, President of the GMC

Although Sir Donald's quote was directed at doctors, it holds good for all clinical professional and support staff and for management within the organisation. Locally, in each of the organisations delivering services to patients, we must strive to ensure that this is how our public measure our services to enable them to feel good about the care they have received, and to help restore the faith that the general public once had in the NHS.

The publication of *The New NHS. Modern. Dependable*[1] heralded a change in the culture through which care is delivered. This is epitomised by two main features:

▶ The importance of team work and partnership

▶ The requirement for rigorous performance management.

Management and organisational structures in NHS Trusts and other organisations already should have changed to reflect these requirements.

The Command Paper,[1] requiring as it does that the quality of care should be the driving force behind the planning of the provision of healthcare, has major implications for staff, given:

▶ public expectations and the need for well-understood and agreed standards for care

▶ staff training and development and re-accreditation

▶ access to information and the greater involvement of staff and patients in the design of the services and their delivery

▶ the development of a culture throughout their services, which allows improvements in patient care to take place.

Additionally, clinical governance requirements arising from the Command Paper[1] will mean that staff:

▶ will have to assume corporate responsibility for the standard and quality of their services

▶ will have to contribute to the development of internal mechanisms for improving clinical performance – identifying quality problems, understanding their causes and acting to bring about improvement, and

▶ will need to understand and develop mechanisms for managing within external mechanisms for improving clinical performance.

Implementing effective clinical governance and improving the quality of services

Crucial to providing high-quality services which can stand up to external scrutiny – including the patients and their carers – and which can change and develop is the right type of culture for the organisation. We hear a great deal about learning organisations, where staff are fully involved in the development of the service and where there is a culture of 'no blame'. Such organisations are appropriately staffed to meet the needs and demands of the patients and have adequate arrangements for cover, study leave, flexible working in order to have a rewarding and sustainable working life. They are creative and anxious to adopt new and better practice; they actually know how they are performing and how they compare with others. They have positive and constructive relationships with partner organisations and do not expend their energies by mindlessly competing with others for organisational gain. They really do share and live a vision relating to the development of top-class patient-focused services, and are flexible and confident enough to embrace all reforms.

It is the Chief Executive who has to lead the process that brings about the change in culture within their organisation to allow them to release the potential of their staff and address constructively the challenges of the future.

Cultural change is never easy and takes a long time and a great deal of effort and commitment on all parties. It involves much listening, communication and action. Cultural change is particularly difficult at the present time, for many of the planks required to effect the necessary changes are not yet in place. There are several reasons for this:

- ▶ Different roles and relationships within the health community have developed with the formation of the Primary Care Trusts, and there have been changes in the role of the Health Authority.

- ▶ Real recruitment difficulties have been experienced by most organisations, which mean that wards and other areas are inadequately staffed and study leave has had to be sacrificed to cover service commitment.

- ▶ Some teams remain incomplete and staffed by temporary occupants.

- ▶ There has been rising patient expectations and a poor press regarding the quality of health services in the country.

- ▶ There has been increasing dependency of patients, and the management of very complex health needs without adequate hospital and primary care resources (in terms of facilities, money and time).

- ▶ Change itself is a factor; it usually paralyses activity for a while.

- ▶ There is a broad range of initiatives to which we expect staff to respond.

A change in culture has to take place in order to manage within the new NHS and really to enable staff to provide the quality and range of service they wish to provide for their patients and which patients wish to receive. The new NHS regimes, and particularly the clinical governance legislation, can provide Chief Executives with the ideal vehicle to remould and change the culture within which they and their staff might work. They can refocus attention on what is really important in the provision of healthcare – namely: the provision of high-quality responsive healthcare through the medium of motivated, well supported, competent and developed staff, well led and managed, in accommodation fit for the purpose.

How, then, can we use clinical governance, not only to allow Chief Executives to meet the goals of the quality strategy, but also to reinforce a sustainable culture for care.

There are a number of elements that Chief Executives have to institute in order to meet these challenges.

Element 1: the process

All organisations have instituted processes through which the quality of clinical care has been measured and monitored in the past. How transparent and accountable these systems have been is questionable, however. There are some high-level performance indicators and some benchmarking information which show whether or not your services differ from others, but audits of all aspects of clinical care have been slow to develop.

Clinical governance and the strategy of quality improvement demand very different processes through which the quality of care can be explicitly described, to the public and internal and external monitoring agencies, and through which Chief Executives can account effectively for the quality of the services in their organisations.

The guidance issued by the Department of Health in *Clinical Governance – Controls Assurance Statements (1999/2000): Risk Management and Organisational Controls*,[3] clearly will help to establish the processes all organisations will require to manage the governance and controls assurance agenda. There are many ways in which the process might be managed. In this chapter, I shall draw on the lessons learned from processes instituted in my own and neighbouring colleagues' NHS Trusts, but I would hasten to warn organisations against setting up a veritable industry through which to manage the process – a particular danger, as clinical governance staff are exempt from management cost controls. Ultimately, a sound and effective process is essential to success – or at least to knowing where an organisation's services rank against approved quality standards. However, it is the *achievement* of those standards that is the important goal we need to reach.

The size and complexity of an organisation's services will be determining factors on the way in which the process of clinical governance and quality improvement is managed. Nevertheless, a comprehensive governance framework must be established to ensure that clinicians and staff throughout the organisation have the opportunity to engage in addressing and implementing the wide range of key targets for clinical governance. The framework needs to encompass:

- clinical audit
- clinical effectiveness
- risk assessment and management (clinical and non-clinical)
- quality assurance
- service improvement
- clinical performance and professional development.

Into this framework must be added public participation and experience and an auditable process to learn from complaints and implement good practice elsewhere.

Essential to the effectiveness of the process is good information and an effective reporting mechanism, which makes the process open and participative and allows staff to develop their services within a culture which is creative, blame-free and informed by validated professional evidence and patients' experiences and views. This is easier said than done. To create the right culture and to institute a robust process requires time and commitment; people have to believe that this is important and that effort must be devoted to it.

All clinicians and staff play a key role in helping the organisation to implement effective clinical governance. All have a responsibility for the standards they achieve in their work; and all need to understand in what framework their individual responsibility and the organisation's responsibility are to be monitored and developed. Communicating well with the staff about these two imperatives is vital. Changing the culture to enable staff to carry out their responsibilities is vital also.

Managers have to be able to answer staff questions about the ways in which these major responsibilities will affect their work. An abstract from the staff information bulletin relating to this issue in North Bristol Trust exemplifies the types of broad questions posed by staff about these dual responsibilities:

> Clinical and Service Standards – recognising the importance of meeting service standards in your workplace
>
> Clinical Audit – fully participating in audit activities and acting on outcomes to improve the services you provide
>
> Risk Management – identifying potential risks or problems in your work and taking action to reduce or prevent problems occurring. Reporting incidents/accidents helps to investigate problems and identify the need for action or resources
>
> Complaints – responding positively to patients' or relatives' concerns and trying to find ways to sort things out to their satisfaction
>
> Quality – looking for opportunities to improve the quality of care or the service you provide, little quality initiatives are just as important as major projects
>
> Performance – working to the best of your abilities and skills, continuing to learn and update your practice, seeking help and advice if you are struggling with any aspect of your work
>
> Raising Concerns – if you have concerns about standards or practices in your workplace, discuss these with colleagues to try and identify solutions or talk to your line manager.
>
> There are clear guidelines for staff regarding their responsibility to raise concerns about standards of care and what to do if these concerns are not listened to or addressed. This is the 'Organisational Openness and Confidentiality Policy' – No. 33 in your Trust handbook of employment policies.[4]

Staff also have to understand the ways in which the organisation itself accounts for its responsibilities, and where their personal accountability fits in to the overall scheme.

Figure 4.1 indicates the way in which the North Bristol NHS Trust has organised the clinical governance process given the large and complex nature of the organisation and its services. The chart looks complex and cumbersome but encompasses all the

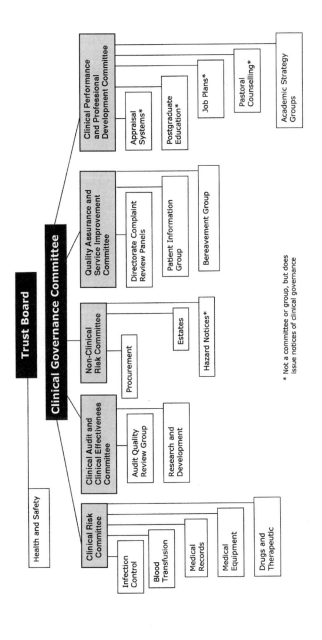

Fig. 4.1. What is the structure for clinical governance at North Bristol NHS Trusts? The Chief Executive has ultimate responsibility for assuring quality of services provided by the Trust. The designated clinicians with executive responsibility for clinical governance are Ms Julie Burgess, Director of Nursing, and Dr Robert Slade, Director. The Clinical Governance Committee has been established as a sub-committee of the board, chaired by a non-executive board member. The committee has responsibility to oversee the development and implementation of clinical governance throughout North Bristol NHS Trust. Dr Peter Simpson, Deputy Medical Director, has responsibility for workforce issues relating to the clinical performance and professional development of medical staff.

elements that require managing and leading in order to have a sound process of accountability and action.

It is vital that staff are kept informed about progress in improving quality within the organisation and the value which the patients, and their carers, place on those improvements.

Presentations, awareness sessions, discussion groups and training on clinical governance issues need to be organised on a regular basis, for clinicians, managers and staff groups. These should to be tailored to the needs of the staff group, highlighting key issues of relevance to their work area.

Additionally, as part of the culture change required, staff must actively be engaged in making improvements to the delivery of care. They frequently complain – rightly – about things that get in the way of delivering a high-quality service. Therefore, as part of this process staff have to be helped to make changes for themselves and not wait for others to make the changes for them. Facilitation is essential where blockages are caused by influences outside their control; however, staff must be empowered to initiate change constructively.

Element 2: Monitoring performance and planning for quality

Everyone working within the NHS will have been aware, in their daily lives, of an increase in the monitoring of everything they do and the outcome of the care they deliver; whether it is the management of their 18-month waiters or the number of days patients within their service stay in hospital following operations. Such data are regularly published in the national newspapers – sometimes in an exceptionally dramatic way – and the league tables are actively debated by press and public alike.

Performance monitoring and management has become an essential element within the day to day operation of any NHS organisation. Currently, much of this monitoring is devoted to the 'absolutely must dos': waiting times and lists, cancelled operations, and so on. However, the performance management systems that have been created to manage these imperatives can be used effectively to place quality at the heart of business planning and strategic development.

Clinical leaders around the country have been involved with their governing bodies in establishing minimum standards for their services. These can be applied universally. They should form part of the monitoring process and allow organisations services to be benchmarked against others.

Additionally, staff and patients should be asked what actually makes a difference to patient care in their services. These elements should be monitored against achievements. This allows staff to feel that they have an influence over the ways in which their services develop, and reinforces the importance of the multidisciplinary team in planning and developing services.

Too frequently in the past, business plans of NHS Trusts comprised filling in holes in finances, or appointing staff to cope with increasing demand, or in catching up with clinical innovation which has not been approved through any recognised process and which suddenly blows a hole through the financial out-turns. Managing the 'here and now' has been to the detriment of standing back and thinking about how services might change and improve, to thinking about doing things differently, to listening to the patients and their relatives about the ways in which care might be delivered, and to accepting that change is really difficult to achieve but is necessary.

If the outcome of clinical governance processes – which include service development based on evidence and examples of good practice – is placed at the heart of the business planning process in the NHS, real quantifiable improvements in patient care might be made that can be underpinned by an effective monitoring system.

The recent staff and public consultation exercise undertaken by the Government has led to the development of those ideas amongst the multidisciplinary teams, which, in turn, is leading to reduced waiting times, better treatment pathways and happier patients and staff. Such initiatives must be underpinned by meaningful staff and public involvement so that organisations can reflect back their innovations in an evaluative framework.

If quality is to be at the core of the strategy for the development of the NHS, we must demonstrate in our planning mechanisms that this is the case, and feed the outcome of the clinical governance process into these mechanisms.

Element 3: Workforce changes, learning environments and appraisal/accreditation systems

Workforce implications and changes

There is no place in the modern NHS for the piecemeal adoption of unproved therapies, or for hanging onto outdated, ineffective treatments. Better guidance is needed on what works for patients and what does not.

Doctors, nurses, midwives and other health professionals, as well as NHS managers and those who commission care, need clear authoritative guidance on where new drugs and therapies best fit beside existing treatments.

The Government's intention is to ensure clear national standards for services, supported by consistent evidence based guidance to raise the quality standards, matching consistency in quality throughout the NHS with sensitivity to the needs of individual patients and local communities.[5]

The Government will help ensure that national quality standards are applied consistently within local practice through a new system of clinical governance; through extending life-long learning to ensure that NHS staff are equipped to deliver change and are given the opportunity to maintain and develop their skills and expertise, and through modernised professional self regulation.[5]

These two statements from the consultative paper – *A First Class Service. Quality in the New NHS*[5] – have significant implications for all staff working in the NHS and especially for the managers, who, for the first time, have a legal accountability and responsibility for the quality of the care offered by the professionals whom they employ.

The implications for the staff are significant:

▶ The public have greater expectations about the quality of care they receive and have a say about the standard of care they actually receive or would wish to receive.

▶ Staff must remain up to date in their clinical practice, as they will be measured publicly on the outcome of the care they provide, and in the future, all medical staff will be re-accredited in order to practice.

▶ Staff must have access to really good quality, easily accessible and relevant information in order to view critically their clinical practice against others.

▶ There will be national guidelines and standards to which all professional staff must sign up and against which they will be measured.

The establishment and monitoring of professional performance and standards will not be a covert 'inhouse' exercise – CHI and the application of National Service Frameworks, accreditation under the Calman Hine arrangements and a new national framework for assessing performance will require all professional staff to be publicly and provably accountable for the outcome of their care, and for Chief Executives to be accountable for the care provided within their organisation.

What does this mean for the professional staff and their managers? There has to be a really well developed relationship between the employer, the regulating professional body, the education provider and the member of staff, to ensure that the necessary professional expertise is available to meet the quality standards and to enable staff to perform effectively (see Figure 4.2 below):

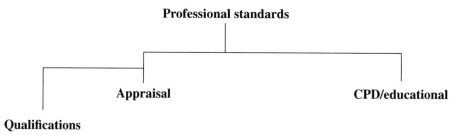

Professional standards

Appraisal   **CPD/educational**

Qualifications

Fig 4.2.   Relationships in organisations practising clinical governance.

This partnership has to exist even before the potential member of staff enters basic training.

The potential employer and the education providers must be clear and explicit about the qualities and competencies sought in potential students in order to aim to enable graduates to be fit for purpose and for practice.

Effective and high-quality healthcare cannot be delivered without having the right people in the right place at the right time, with the right skills to care for patients.

This means that the NHS has to become much clearer about the competencies they require from their staff members, and overall workforce planning must improve.

All this requires a cultural change for both the professionals working within the services, their relationships with their employers, and for those involved in the relationship between the providers of education and training, the regulatory bodies and health service employers.

The ways in which healthcare is changing are many. The requirements for health service employers and their professional staff to meet the requirements of the quality frameworks places an increasing need on the employers to assure the quality of the care provided by individuals and teams and to provide the necessary continuing professional development (CPD) for their staff. The consequences for the four partners are set out below.

▶ *Employers* will have to ensure that there is a continuous check kept on the ways in which staff are developing to ensure that they maintain the competence and relevance of the staff they employ. They will have to have in place appropriate appraisal and assessment systems, based on good clinical standards and best clinical practice, and they will have to commit themselves to providing CPD for their professional staff.

▶ *Professional staff* will have to commit themselves to being regularly appraised and assessed, to providing only care which is evidence-based and audited; they will have to be more flexible in their approach to their post as the care which they are likely to give patients will change dramatically over the lifetime of their work and they have to change and adapt themselves with it. There are no jobs for life anymore.

▶ *Purchasers of education* will have to ensure that the organisations on whose behalf they commission education have good workforce planning models in place, that education is commissioned on a competency-based model, and that flexibility is built into the contracts with the providers of education. Their specification of the educational requirements must be accurate and ensure that the resultant 'graduates' are fit for purpose and practice. Whenever possible, staff should be trained in teams – for that is how they are required to work.

▶ *Providers of education* will have to ensure that they understand and appreciate the needs of the service for competent staff, that they enter into a positive relationship with their purchasers and work with them to deliver the workforce for the future.

There is a lot of work to be done together but the quality agenda will not be achieved unless the essential partnership between employer, professional body and education provider is consolidated and improved.

Learning environments
In order to establish this synergy between the employer, the trainers and the staff, and develop a constructive learning environment, a truly creative learning environment must be provided.

Traditionally, often there has been a somewhat tense relationship between employers and their staff-side representatives. The direction given within *The New NHS. Modern. Dependable*,[1] however, points to a more creative and supportive relationship between the employers in the NHS and their staff and staff representatives. This is clearly sensible and should enable there to be an improvement in the ways in which care can and is delivered. If industrial models are used that have successfully transformed this vital relationship, much progress may be made. All staff have to be employed in reducing waste, in challenging outcome and methods of working and creating the clear shared goal towards which the organisation is moving.

Such dynamic relationships are underpinned by an understanding of evidence-based practice and its monitoring and a full and creative relationship with 'customers'. Practice must be underpinned by training that takes place in an environment in which it is safe to admit errors and take the necessary action to correct faults. The organisations that evolve are characterised by reward and acknowledgement, a very creative environment, low turnover, real opportunities for promotion and the recognition of, and best use of, talent.

A great deal of debate has surrounded the learning environment and life-long learning in the NHS and the role it will play in the successful implementation of clinical governance regimes in the NHS. The environment and resource needs that are to be created before this concept will become much more than words. If NHS organisations do not take action to create such a culture for the future, we shall never hold on to our good staff or recruit enthusiastic replacements. Nothing destroys the quality of the services provided by the NHS faster than a service provided by temporary staff so that teams can never be created and develop together.

Appraisal and effective review processes

The establishment of effective review processes is essential to the clinical governance agenda. Clear standards are under development in all the medical colleges and nursing regulators to govern the standards of care to be expected from a qualified and registered practitioner. However, the methodology through which those standards are attained, and the nature of CPD accompanying this, are, as yet, unclear, although the GMC document[6] clearly highlights the absolute requirement for formal assessment and performance review against those standards in the future.

Many professions have been undertaking appraisal and assessment for many years, but the outcome has infrequently been available publicly.

It seems ineffective, in driving forward a team-based approach to improving quality of service and outcome for patients for the various professions, to have different appraisal and accreditation systems so that accounting for the quality of the service as well as the practitioner is nullified. Good assessment processes are essential in maintaining and improving the quality of services. An understanding of the terms that 'float' around this process clearly also are essential.

An evaluated pilot of appraisal of consultant medical staff[7] has just been completed, and it is essential to have a clear and shared understanding of the use of terminology in the report.

The definitions the team involved in the pilot have used so far are set out below.

1. Appraisal: The prime purpose is developmental. It must include a review of the professional's revalidation action folder and be a continuous record of practice.
2. Performance management: The prime purpose is managerial. It ensures that the individual is meeting contractual, departmental and organisational objectives and standards.
3. Revalidation: The prime purpose is professional self-regulation. It ensures fitness to practice against standards of safety and professional competence.

Additional to these, the following subset of definitions was agreed:

▶   Appraisal is primarily an educational/development process for the purpose of reviewing the appraisee's performance over a range of areas and a period of time. It is pastoral, not punitive.

▶   Assessment is for the purposes of judging and then regulating performance according to a set of external professional standards. Its function is career regulation rather than education.[8]

The content of appraisal can be translated well into the more regulatory requirements for assessment and re-accreditation. To develop the appraisal process, the study[7] found that the following were required:

▶   A peer review model, including defining the purpose, aims and outcomes

▶   Development of appraisal content

▶   An appraisal structure

▶   Documentation

▶   An interview structure

▶   Identification of skills

▶   Training in the structure, skills and application

▶   Evaluation.

The evidence emerging from the first round of pilot peer appraisals in this region indicates that the process is regarded, by the vast majority of participating doctors, as very helpful and supportive. Whilst some concern has been expressed about managing the poor performers, the steering group for the pilot appraisal project felt that their priority was to develop a system that was motivating, helpful and beneficial to the 90% of all practising hospital doctors whose performance falls well within acceptable performance levels. The mechanisms for dealing with those few who may not want to benefit from the process also have been put in place.

Whilst the outputs, in terms of development plans, may, on the surface, seem obvious and not particularly noteworthy, the effort that went into supporting and encouraging individuals to pursue their needs indicates that a fundamental requirement is being met. This model of peer review was designed to be of benefit to the appraisee; the post-appraisal questionnaire data support an overall positive shift in perception, even after limited exposure to appraisal.

The summary of the published report[7] into the appraisal methodology and outcome stated:

> Peer review is an effective feedback mechanism that reviews performance (appraisal), allows for the identification of strengths (motivating) and those areas needing development (risk management). From this plans are formed, resources for development needs identified and schedules set (development). Thus we propose that the purpose of performance appraisal for senior doctors will encapsulate these same key ingredients: appraisal, motivation, risk management, development and assessment. This will ensure an effective and reliable process for supporting the personal and professional development of senior doctors.

Wallace summarises in his article[9] that Trust Executives and Health Authorities underestimate the tasks ahead in relation to emerging policies on clinical governance. Sponsoring the development of peer review in the South West has provided the opportunity for a more accurate analysis of the future costs and resource implications of at least one requirement of clinical governance – an effective review process.

The outcome of the report was a valuable methodology, as well as a better understanding of the time that needs to be devoted to undertaking such exercises – an additional cost to providing a quality service.

The ways in which poor performers might be dealt with constructively, but with determination, emerged from the exercise. Peer appraisal, albeit a developmental undertaking, allows poor performance to be identified and reported on – through the failure to sign off a candidate's appraisal. It then lies with the Medical Director to invoke the appropriate formal mechanisms through which he and the Chief Executive can manage the poor performance of any individual in an organisation, in line with policies and practices agreed within the organisation.

Element 4: Good information – acting on results

Without good information, a Chief Executive will have no idea about the quality of care provided by practitioners in his or her organisation. Clinical indicators and clinical benchmarking data provide useful guidance on the information required to monitor the quality of a service delivered by a team; but an in-depth understanding is needed if credit is to be given to exceptional performance or if action needs to be taken to make up for any deficiencies. Quality monitoring must be given equal status in performance management to achieve the goal of knowing the outcome of care.

To achieve this, information systems are needed which are accurate and allow evaluation of outcomes and which can be managed within a monitoring and accountability framework. This in turn must:

▶ give explicit foci of accountability

▶ provide clear definitions

▶ measure processes

▶ have explicit and correct data

▶ have robust control mechanisms

▶ be managed via sensitive central management

▶ monitor down to ward or unit level, and

▶ be clear about risk assessment.

Integral to acting on the outcome of the performance management systems must be a real and provable ability to learn from experience and to avoid the lessons highlighted by failure. The recently published guidance from the Chief Medical Officer, *An Organisation with a Memory*,[10] clearly outlines the importance of the whole service learning from mistakes and also from the experience of patients. There is little purpose in providing a faultless service in the future if this proves to be a service not liked or helpful to the people for whom it is provided.

The embedding of the views of the patient in clinical governance and thus the quality of the service in an organisation is critical – and fits in well with the themes of better and more empowered staff involvement. How to gain this information and use it effectively is quite difficult, however.

Supporting the redesign of care around the patient is a key theme in the new *NHS Plan: A Plan for Investment; A Plan for Reform*:[11]

> Patients are the most important people in the health service. It doesn't always appear that way. Too many patients feel talked at, rather than listened to. This has to change. NHS care has to be shaped around the convenience and concerns of patients. To bring this about, patients must have more say in their own treatment and more influence over the way the NHS works. The reforms outlined here give patients new rights and new roles within the health service.

Through the initiatives outlined in this report,[11] patients will receive better information which will empower them to better look after their own health and know about their local health services and the treatment planned for them. The NHS will have to get used to being scrutinised publicly and will have to act now to ensure that it learns all lessons from the information available to it through the patient experience, through peer review outcomes and through clinical indicators.

Summary

The theme running through the *NHS Plan: A Plan for Treatment; A Plan for Reform*[11] is clear – it underpins the strategy outlined in *The New NHS. Modern. Dependable*[1] that the quality of care delivered is to become the driving force for the development of health services. The *NHS Plan: A Plan for Treatment; A Plan for Reform*[11] makes it clear that the NHS will ensure that services are driven by a cycle of continuous quality improvement. Quality will not be restricted just to the clinical aspects of care, but will include quality of life and the entire patient experience. Healthcare organisations and professions will establish ways to identify procedures that should be modified or abandoned, and will develop new practices that lead to improved patient care. All those providing care will work to make it ever safer, and support a culture where we can learn from, and effectively reduce, mistakes. The NHS will continuously improve its efficiency, productivity and performance.

At a very minimum, all Chief Executives should now have in place an active and meaningful response to and future action plan for the introduction of clinical governance in their organisations, as required by the Health Service Commissioner. This must comprise the following:

▶ competent clinical audit

▶ systems of regular appraisal for all staff and systems, policies and procedures to identify and deal with poor performance

▶ a forum to assess evidence-based developments

▶ a responsible approach to clinical cost-effectiveness

▶ evidence of seeking feedback on patient experience, and evidence that the service responds to that feedback

▶ a management structure to address clinical governance and quality in the context of performance management, and

▶ the understanding of the board and its executives and managers about the quality of services provided.

Added to this, the themes that emerge from making the quality of services fundamental to all activities allow the Chief Executive a variety of really exciting opportunities to mould and change, if necessary, the culture of the organisation, to revitalise staff and patient involvement and to deliver an organisation which achieves and is responsive, keen and motivated.

References

1 Department of Health. *The New NHS. Modern. Dependable.* Command paper 3807. London: Department of Health, December 1997.
2 Department of Health. *Clinical Governance: Quality in the New NHS.* London: Department of Health. Health Service Commissioner 1999/065. March 1999.
3 Department of Health. *Governance in the NHS: Controls Assurance Statements (1999/2000): Risk Management and Organisational Controls.* London: Department of Health. HSC 1999/123, May 1999.
4 Department of Health. Organisational openness and confidentiality policy, No. 33 in Trust Handbook of Employment Policies, in accordance with EL (93) 51 *Guidance for Staff on Relations with the Public and Media.* London: Department of Health, 1993.
5 Department of Health. *A First Class Service. Quality in the New NHS.* Consultation document on quality in the new NHS. HSC 1998/113. Wetherby: Department of Health, July 1998.
6 General Medical Council. *Performance Procedures.* London: General Medical Council, July 1997.
7 Lloyd S, Hasler J, Smith P. *Peer Review: What's In It For Me?* Edgcumbe Consulting, 2000.
8 Jolly B, Grant J. *The Good Assessment Guide.* Joint Centre for Education in Medicine, 1997.

9   Wallace L. When the buck stops here: Perspectives from the top of health authorities and trusts in the West Midlands on clinical governance and evidence based-medicine. *Proceedings of the British Psychological Society* 2000; 8(1)3.

10   Department of Health. *An Organisation with a Memory.* Report of an expert group on learning from adverse events in the NHS. London: Department of Health, 2000.

11   The Rt Hon. Alan Milburn, MP Secretary of State for Health. *NHS Plan: A Plan for Investment; A Plan for Reform.* London: Department of Health, July 2000.

Nursing and Midwifery Contribution to Clinical Governance

Anna Maslin

As I reflected on why I had been asked to write this chapter, a number of thoughts came to mind. Like many of my nursing and midwifery colleagues, I have a number of roles and have had numerous experiences in our healthcare service. In my own case, this has encompassed being a professional, working as a clinician, an educator, a manager and a researcher, but it also has encompassed being a patient, a patient's daughter, a mother, wife and friend. I experienced maternity services for the first time while working as a student nurse 21 years ago, then as an expectant mother 14 years ago and again as a later mother only two years ago. Like colleagues and patients, I have experienced first hand the dilemmas, challenges and improvements that have developed in healthcare.

In my professional life, I specialised in oncology. We worked consistently to improve cancer services; to ensure patients were treated as individuals and had quality information; to ensure patients had choice and were supported; to ensure the physical and psychological assaults of disease and treatment were minimised; and to ensure that patients were treated by a specialist multidisciplinary team. These efforts were rewarded, and what started as a mission of the few became an unstoppable movement. I would never claim we have arrived, but there have been significant improvements in cancer care and, as a result, there are an army of professional and lay colleagues who continue to take the challenge forward.

In the field of quality, nurses and midwives often have led the way, working with patients and other professionals to deliver the highest possible standards of care. This commitment and valuable input to quality was highlighted in the nursing, midwifery and health visiting strategy document *Making a Difference*. In my view, nurses and midwives are uniquely placed to deliver quality improvements where they are most needed – at the direct interface with the patient. There is no reason why this should change. Certainly, the agenda has been refocused and an urgency brought to modernising the NHS, but the principles remain the same: to provide high-quality healthcare to patients which is responsive, provided equitably and is focused on the key issues facing our NHS.

Some nurses and midwives may have been given the impression that clinical governance is a medical preserve, but this is patently not the case; clinical governance is about patients. It is about providing quality services to patients in a spirit of true partnership. Partnership between nurses, midwives, doctors, the multidisciplinary team, but more importantly between patients and the NHS is vital. It is about creating a culture where true collaboration takes place and services are provided that meet patients' needs and expectations while at the same time allowing health professionals, including nurses and midwives, to deliver the best care they are capable of. Clinical governance is 'a framework through which the NHS organisations are accountable for continuously improving the quality of their services and safeguarding high standards of care, by creating an environment in which excellence in clinical care will flourish'.

It is imperative that all professionals are engaged in this process. Nurses and midwives, in particular, have so much to contribute to the development of clinical governance, as they are so often at the forefront of quality innovation.

Nurses and midwives should be involved in setting up the framework for clinical governance in their particular clinical area. The scope of their responsibilities obviously will vary depending on their role within the organisation, and their organisation will have set up lines of accountability and responsibility. Work should have been done to establish a baseline assessment and a development plan that is designed to take the work forward.

Now that the Chief Executive has a statutory responsibility for the quality of care in a NHS provider, the focus on quality is acute. There now should be a culture where nurses' and midwives' concerns regarding the improvement of the quality of care for patients is welcomed. In day to day terms, the lead for advancing clinical governance can be taken by a senior clinician, usually at board level. It could be a Medical Director, but now, very frequently, it is taken on by the Director of Nursing, leading to a title of 'Director of Nursing/Quality'. Local commissioning groups currently are setting up their own arrangements for clinical governance but, again, in a number of cases nurses and midwives are taking the lead, sometimes in cooperation with a GP.

The NHS provider's development plan is a fundamental document that nurses and midwives should participate actively in producing and monitoring. It is important that nurses and midwives at all levels know who is the lead for clinical governance in their area. Moreover, it is important nurses and midwives are aware of, and are participating in, the practical steps to ensure clinical governance is a success.

For nurses and midwives, there must be:

▶ The recognition that every member of staff in the multidisciplinary team has a unique role in the provision of high-quality care to their patients and clients.

▶ The understanding that clinical governance is about improving the quality of care using the most appropriate methods. The process involves the identification of the problem, an assessment of the situation, a structured plan for improvement, monitoring of that plan and evaluation of the outcome to ensure future plans for improvement are informed by evidence.

▶ The understanding that clinical governance is about being accountable for your care to the wider world. Colleagues, patients and the public all want to be safe in the knowledge that they are receiving the most appropriate and skilful care possible.

▶ The understanding that the systems nurses and midwives work in must be assessed to ensure they are enabling them to work to the best of their ability.

Poor physical conditions or poor organisation all can impact on our ability to provide the best care we are capable of.

Case study

Sister Ann Taylor had just taken up a new post in a major trauma accident and emergency department. After working around the clock to get a feel for the department, she became conscious that, although the numbers of nursing colleagues for staffing were adequate, there were patients waiting for substantial periods to see the senior house officer (SHO) at night. She noted the frustrations of patients and nursing staff who had to wait for a medical discharge even for minor injuries. These patients often became irritated and, as a result, a proportion of them were taking their own discharge against advice. Other patients with more complex injuries often had to wait longer than she felt acceptable and once again the nursing staff felt powerless to improve the situation.

Ann was aware of the onus on her and all her colleagues to improve the situation, and, as a result, she had an informal conversation with the main accident and emergency consultant, Barbara Sims, and made an appointment to come and discuss the situation further with her. Once they had shared their concerns, Ann agreed to take the lead in conducting a baseline assessment to help them identify the strengths and weaknesses of the care they were providing. They agreed to share their thoughts and discussions at the multidisciplinary team meeting the following week.

The rest of the team were feeling somewhat hesitant about the proposed exercise but could see the potential value to the patients and to the rest of the staff. Ann and Barbara reassured them that once the baseline information was available, they would bring it back to the team meeting and share with them how the information related to their local Health Improvement Programmes and National Service Frameworks before they decided to go any further.

As Ann was the lead for this initial assessment, she decided, as part of the overall piece of work, to conduct a SWOT (Strengths, Weaknesses, Opportunities and potential Threats) analysis in the department. She asked as many of the staff who were willing to contribute their thoughts and observations, including the junior doctors, who felt, not unnaturally, that they were being unjustly made the focus of attention.

Ann adopted another approach to get her baseline information: she conducted a significant-event audit. She chose this method because she felt it would be a reasonably straightforward way to look at a difficult situation. Ann brought together a cross section of the staff and shared with them one of the incidents which sparked her initial concerns.

At about 02:00 hours, Ann had been doing her rounds in the department and had noticed a 70-year-old woman in one of the cubicles with her daughter beside her. The lady's name was Mrs Davis, and it appeared she had fallen down a flight of stairs just before midnight. After her fall, Mrs Davis managed to crawl to a telephone to ring her daughter, who came straight around and called an ambulance. The ambulance arrived about 00:30 hours and Mrs Davis was admitted to the department at around 01:00 hours with suspected head or neck fractures, or both.

Mrs Davis clearly was in pain and acutely distressed at being secured in a neck and body brace. The department was reasonably busy but there were adequate numbers of nursing staff present. The main limiting factor to Mrs Davis receiving prompt attention was the fact that only one casualty officer was available at that time. Mrs Davis – who was in significant pain – was not seen by a doctor until 03:30 hours. She and her daughter were polite but it was obvious that they were not at all happy with the situation.

The nurses felt guilty and helpless, and, as a result, they didn't go into the cubicle more often than was necessary. This avoidance on their part seemed to make the situation worse for them, as well as for the patient and her daughter, who felt even more isolated.

Once Mrs Davis was seen by the SHO, and a X-ray was requested, it was a further two hours before the results were conveyed to her, pain relief obtained and the brace removed. Mrs Davis had a fracture to her spine but her head and upper neck were unaffected by the fall.

Mrs Davis was finally admitted to her ward at 08:00 hours.

Ann asked the team to identify the key issues in this significant event. In their view, the key components were as follows:

▶ Medical staffing

▶ Feelings of impotence due to role limitations

▶ Pain control protocols

▶ Communication and psychological support – provision for patients and staff.

The team then discussed each area in turn using the simple SWOT formula to look creatively at solutions for improving the care of other patients in a similar situation.

Once Ann had gathered the data, she and Barbara met to discuss the findings. They realised very quickly that there was an issue with medical staffing, which Barbara would pursue with the Medical Director, but there also was an issue about nursing and the very high level of education and skills the nurses now possessed. Together, they agreed that Ann should discuss this with her Nurse Executive Director to explore the options open to them to extend practice.

Ann and Barbara shared the information gathered, and outlined their suggestions for the next steps. The team was interested but hesitant. The nursing staff could see the possibilities that a review might lead to and became quite enthusiastic. The medical staff felt reassured that they were being offered support rather than criticism, but some of the support staff were concerned that any change may negatively impact on their workload.

The team together decided that they would review the Trust's guidelines and take positive steps to generally take this work on quality forward. They decided they should look at a number of other areas, including the following:

▶ Risk management

▶ Development of information systems

▶ Review of medical audit procedures

▶ Review of nursing audit procedures

▶ Review of significant-event audit procedures

▶ Strategic plans for professional development

▶ Current objectives for the department.

As a department, they realised someone would need to take the lead on implementing this new way of working and thinking in relation to clinical governance. One of the lecturer practitioners, Liz Hurley, felt that she would like to take the lead role as part of her ongoing professional development, provided she had the full support of Ann and Barbara and the genuine cooperation of the rest of the staff.

Liz decided to identify and meet the Trust's lead person for clinical governance, as well as to seek out other locally available sources of general information and support. She decided also to initiate meetings with other departments to identify their lead person for clinical governance so that she could learn from their experiences so far.

Once the initial baseline assessment was completed and the initial plans for action implemented, Ann was content that the department was on its way to making a positive start. She and Barbara felt the department was committed to the clinical governance approach, and she felt sure that everyone realised their crucial contribution to making it happen.

The team agreed to work with Liz to ensure their departmental priorities fitted into the Trust's priorities and that they were dovetailed into local priorities included in their local Health Improvement Programmes, as well as into national priorities such as the National Service Frameworks.

As an accident and emergency department, they were aware that the national work on antibiotic prescribing, cancer services, mental health services and coronary heart disease would impact on them and the care they needed to provide to their patients.

As our case study noted, nurses and midwives need to be aware of the sources of support and information available to them (for example, NHS guidelines, professional organisation guidelines, clinical guidelines, systematic reviews and clinical research) to enable them to fulfil their responsibilities. There is also now a NHS Clinical Governance Support Team. This multiprofessional team, led by Professor Aidan Halligan, will help nurses and midwives to implement clinical governance in a practical way. The key nurse on the team is Catherine Elcoat. The team will work directly with the NHS to support progress on clinical governance by empowering staff to make change at the local level. Its work will be profession-friendly and patient-centred. It will aim to provide practical support, through a helpline, for NHS staff, through worked-up models of clinical governance in practice, and by focusing on leadership development. The team is there to work with everyone – including nurses and midwives – to help us all overcome barriers to progress.

Having systems like those outlined above is fundamental to enable us to create a healthcare system that is consistent and equitable; but to achieve this, we must have the commitment of everyone working within an organisation. Every nurse and midwife has a part to play – as part of an organisation, as a professional and as an individual. As nurses and midwives, our role is different from that of a doctor or any other professional caring for patients. We are in the unique position of being well placed to influence colleagues and patients alike. We are clearly a professional group which spans all healthcare environments from primary to acute care. Already, we are very comfortable with working within a multiagency environment. We have long promoted the concept of team working but nurses and midwives need support too. It is crucial that there is strong leadership in place, that continuing professional development is seen as vital and that appropriate information is continuously shared.

Good care depends on effective collaboration between many people. How those people work together is a crucial determinant of the quality of care. Within teams and when working on our own, nurses and midwives bring a unique contribution to the quality of care and more specifically to clinical governance. Nurses and midwives have a central place within any multidisciplinary team; often, they are the only point of regular contact in a patient's care. Other professionals will become involved in their care at different times, but in many cases the nurse or midwife will be there throughout, which gives them a perspective that is invaluable. They can see where the interface between professionals and different organisations works well and, more importantly, where it is *not* working well. Clinical governance spans the artificial barriers created by professions and organisations. It needs to follow the patients – to be patient-centred. Our insights need to be fed into the review of services, to ensure that change creates seamless care for the patient – whether they are receiving their care from nurses, midwives, doctors or therapists. The following case report is a good example of this.

Mr James is a 56-year-old professional man with T-cell chronic lymphocytic leukemia (TCLL). He is often neutropeanic and anaemic. Mr James had been a chronic leukaemic for 12 years when he started to require blood transfusions every two weeks. During this period, he also started to pick up very severe infections which could leave him unconscious very rapidly. Mr James's wife was obviously very frightened but she was reassured by the oncology team caring for him. Her main difficulty was the fact that she could tell when he was becoming acutely ill but, because it all happened so quickly and she couldn't drive, she was always in the position of having to call an ambulance. The ambulance would come and often some time would elapse before Mr James was admitted to the oncology ward where the nurses and doctors knew him.

Staff nurse Vince Hall realised the situation was causing Mr and Mrs James a great deal of concern, and he spoke to colleagues, who agreed with him that admission protocols needed updating particularly for patients like Mr James. As a team, they did a piece of work looking at streamlining the service that chronic oncology patients experienced, and set to work to ensure that everyone within and outside the department was aware of the new arrangements.

Vince discussed the new arrangements with Mr and Mrs James and made sure their

GP was content. In the future, all Mrs James has to do is call an ambulance and let the ward know her husband is on his way in when she felt his condition was deteriorating. With the new system, admission formalities were bypassed until Mr James was safely on the ward, where immediate treatment and care could be started.

Nursing and midwifery professionals have always been at the forefront of involving patients and their carers in the planning and delivery of clinical care. Their unique position can engender strong and trusting relationships with patients and families, and so create a unique opportunity to influence service provision so that it better meets patient need and expectation.

Nurses and midwives often have been involved in undertaking research to establish the views of patients and carers in many specialities. Research can focus on providing an evidence base to help us look for ways to improve care but also to identifying problems. In our illustration above, Ann chose to use a significant-event audit as a tool to gathering her baseline information; but other options are possible. Problems can be identified by:

▶ encouraging free and open communication

▶ providing staff with supportive clinical supervision

▶ conducting a needs assessment

▶ monitoring all letters of complaint or praise regularly, and looking out for recurring themes or issues

▶ surveying patients

▶ using quality, published research to compare the results or recommendations with current practice, and

▶ conducting a formal research study subject to scientific and Ethics Committee approval.

At one time, it was very easy to see a patient as a series a symptoms – a puzzle to be solved, an illness to be cured. But patients are more than that. Nurses and midwives are very good at seeing patients as human beings that need both care *and* cure (if possible). This care may be much wider than the direct treatment of a set of symptoms. This perspective and a focus on caring is, I believe, a fundamental strength of nurses, midwives and health visitors. We need to see beyond the symptoms to the patient and work to provide care to them in a comprehensive and cohesive way. There is no point in X-raying an elderly woman for a fracture, reassuring her all is well, then discharging her in the middle of the night to an empty flat.

Throughout the country, health visitors, whilst encouraging and enabling young families to make full use of developmental and health screening services, also concentrate on helping young people to become confident parents by teaching them parenting skills and putting them in touch with voluntary and statutory organisations. They may, for example, need help in accessing Social Services to sort out a housing problem, or they may need to be introduced to the school nurse who will be able to assist the older child who has been having problems settling into his/her new class. By taking this holistic approach, health visitors are stretching their role and therefore their accountability, which requires them to be fully aware at all times of their responsibilities within set regulations.

Evaluation of nurse-led services demonstrates that because nurses are in contact with the patient longer than are doctors, they are able to discuss more fully the range of options open to patients. Advising patients and their families is an increasingly important part of the professional role, as is making sound, evidence-based information available to them and actively supporting their choices so that the patients themselves are participants in, not merely recipients of, healthcare. Information and information technology are valuable assets in this process.

The nursing and midwifery professions regularly uses operational clinical systems to extract and analyse information; for example:

▶ to identify patients suffering from a particular condition or to measure the incidence of pressure sores

▶ to assess compliance with treatment protocols in line with National Service Frameworks

▶ to check compliance with monitoring processes to manage and avoid long-term complications, and

▶ to monitor outcomes of care.

Moreover, an increasingly wide range of material will become available – for example, through the NHS Net and the Electronic Library for Health.

Nurses must use evidence-based information to inform their practice, and to communicate information to their patients so that they are engaged actively in decisions about their healthcare.

As medicine has advanced, many of the treatments offered to patients have become more and more complex. It is easy in such areas to lose sight of what the care is intended to do – to improve the health of the patient. In many cases, treatment has grown incrementally as time has gone by, and new ways of delivering elements of care have been developed. Often, there is a need to step back from the detail and look at the big picture. We need to ensure that the appropriate professional delivers services in the most clinically effective way, in the most suitable setting. Because nurses and midwives are in contact with patients for prolonged periods of time, they are able to tease out the likely concerns that patients have and ensure that services are developed in such a way as to reflect their individual needs.

Benchmarking techniques are being used increasingly by groups of practitioners to structure the comparison and sharing of examples of good practice to address patients concerns about the quality of nursing care (eg complaints about not being washed, not being fed, not being treated with respect, etc). Benchmarks of best practice are identified by patients and professionals as a means of identifying the essential elements of high-quality care and this provides important information on which to establish an improvement-based approach to clinical practice and service delivery. The NHS Executive is establishing regional support networks for clinical benchmarking activity. Regional facilitators will assist in establishing comparison groups of practitioners who then can use the benchmarks to identify action plans that will ensure practice is shared and developed to consistently achieve high-quality care.

We have considered some of the ways nurses and midwives can contribute to the clinical governance agenda. Clinical governance will lead to exciting changes in the way services are delivered. The role of nurses and midwives is changing and we need to ensure that this continues to enable the new challenges ahead to be met. We are already beginning to see this happening in many of the key initiatives (NHS Direct, walk-in centres, etc.) within the NHS (discussed below).

NHS Direct

NHS Direct,[2] the nurse-led service, puts nursing firmly at the forefront of the drive to develop more accessible and responsive healthcare. It aims to provide prompt access to professional advice and reassurance 24 hours a day, 365 days a year. It can enable patients to care for themselves at home or directs them quickly to the right service, at the right time. NHS Direct aims to empower patients to take greater control of their own health and well being.

It is clearly an innovation that works to benefit patients, but also it opens exciting and challenging opportunities for nurses – to make better use of their knowledge and skills and to build on these skills in a dynamic environment, and to take the lead in developing a service that provides the very best of care and support to patients and their families.

NHS Direct is an example of how nursing professionals can make a difference by working in partnership with patients.

Walk-in centres

All walk-in centres are nurse-led and they provide another unique opportunity. The services provided by these centres aim to enable the public to make informed choices about their own health and to encourage them to use services in the appropriate way. Centres will provide a range of services, including advice about self care, healthy lifestyles, and management of minor ailments and injuries. They will also direct people to other health services – both statutory and voluntary – often in conjunction with NHS Direct. They should be conveniently located and open at times that suit modern lifestyles, and they are intended to compliment existing primary care centres.

Nurses and midwives will need to work flexibly and will need to be adaptable in order to respond appropriately to user requirements. We will need to continue to recognise the importance of diversity and the need to respect the right of users to exercise their choice. In particular, we will have to ensure that the information we provide is up-to-date and communicated in a responsible, relevant and timely way.

New roles for nurses in primary care

The new primary care agenda has enabled nurses to consider new roles, particularly in the development of Primary Care Groups and Trusts. Nurses will have an important influence over decisions about service development

At a clinical level, nurse prescribing has offered the opportunity for over 25 000 nurses with a district nursing or health visiting qualification to be trained to prescribe from the nurse prescribing formulary by March 2001. Furthermore, in the future, district nurses and health visitors completing their community specialist practitioner qualification also will be qualified as nurse prescribers.

Throughout the country, practice nurses are now essential members of primary care teams, leading the way in running clinics and providing expert support to patients and expert advice to professional colleagues.

For patients, nurse involvement in key roles in primary care and in building integrated care pathways provides a more consistent and effective approach to healthcare delivery – one that works and one that patients trust. From the nurses' perspective, it enhances our role, giving us opportunities to take on new responsibilities and to be truly accountable for the quality of service provided.

Nurse consultants

Nurse consultants are now a reality, and working at this level will challenge post-holders to accumulate, coherently and effectively, knowledge and expertise related to an area of practice. They will need to apply new knowledge to their own and others' practice in structured ways which can be evaluated, as well as interpret and evaluate information from diverse sources to make informed judgements about its quality and appropriateness.

Nurse consultants have the opportunity to monitor actively the effectiveness of current therapeutic programmes and integrate different aspects of practice, to improve outcomes for patients and clients, whilst managing constantly changing scenarios in the interest of patients and clients.

Key to their role is promotion of the improvement of quality and clinical effectiveness within resource constraints. In order to do this, they will have to assess and monitor continuously risk in their own and others' practice, as well as challenge others about wider risk factors. An essential element of the Nurse consultants being able to achieve this will be their ability to evaluate and audit continually their own practice and that of others. This involves applying a broad range of valid and reliable evaluation methods, as well as utilising critical appraisal skills to analyse the outcomes of research evaluations and audits, and apply them to improve practice.

Whichever way we look, nurses and midwives are demonstrating their wide-ranging ability to be full members of the healthcare team, taking clinical governance forward in partnership with patients and clients. The expertise nurses and midwives undoubtedly have will help to improve services. As nurses and midwives, we must build consistently on current excellence, as well as constantly identify and rectify poorer performance as part of our corporate responsible within our organisations. Nurses and midwives have a significant contribution to make to the clinical governance agenda and I am confident we will be seen to be making it.

The views expressed in this chapter are personal and all names in the case studies are fictitious.

Bibliography

Department of Health. *A First Class Service: Quality in the New NHS*. London, 1998.

Department of Health. *Making a Difference. Strengthening the Nursing, Midwifery and Health Visiting Contribution to Health and Healthcare*. London, 1999.

Roland M, Baker R. *Clinical Governance. A Practical Guide for Primary Care Teams*. Manchester: University of Manchester, 1999.

Royal College of Nursing. *Clinical Governance: How Nurses Can Get Involved*. London, 2000.

www.nhsdirect.nhs.uk; 0845 4647.

▶6

Role of the Medical Director

Jenny Simpson

> *'The Medical Director is the guardian of clinical probity': Dr Alastair Scotland, Medical Directors Group, The British Association of Medical Managers, October 1993.*

The complex and constantly evolving role of the Medical Director provides a fascinating perspective from which to view the development of clinical governance. The Medical Director in any NHS organisation is so closely involved in the development of clinical governance, it could perhaps be said that the principles of clinical governance more or less define the job of the Medical Director.

This chapter sets out to examine the role of the Medical Director – perhaps the most challenging position in today's NHS. First, the context is set, by exploring the development of the role from the beginning, moving on to discuss the nature of the job and the practical realities that face the Medical Director. An analysis of the turbulent environment of the NHS follows, and the chapter concludes with a discussion of the skills and knowledge Medical Directors need to be able to do the job. The underlying thesis is that in most organisations the Medical Director is the key player in clinical governance. It is crucial for the long-term health of the NHS that Medical Directors have the highest level of education and development, as well as sophisticated support systems, so that they are equipped to deliver these complex and challenging roles, in an ever-changing environment, effectively and with confidence.

The early days

When Trusts were first created, following the 1991 white paper *Working for Patients,*[1] the uniting feature of the job was a singular lack of clarity. The white paper had positioned the Medical Director as a statutory role, but the nature of the job was neither described nor defined. The ethos of the day was to let Trusts find their own way of developing the role, and, as a result, the job very much reflected the culture of the Trust itself.

Job descriptions – and indeed contracts – were either vague or entirely absent, and for the first two years or so, each Medical Director's job was peculiar to the individual organisation. Medical Directors largely assumed that the role was representative, providing the medical staff view at the Trust board. At board meetings in the early days of Trusts, Medical Directors functioned very much as the former chairmen of medical staff committees and adopted much the same behaviour.

Early on, there were Medical Directors in post with no specific time allocated and no reward whatsoever. In reality, these individuals were regarded as mere figureheads with no real managerial influence to speak of. Over the first few months, many Medical Directors fell by the wayside, as it became clear that not only was the role extremely complex, but also that it demanded a great deal from the busy clinician.

As the months went by, it became very clear that the role of the medical director had a number of different aspects. A striking phenomenon in the early days was the variation between Medical Director jobs – one Medical Director spent most of his management time finding beds for acute emergency admissions, whilst another was solely concerned with sorting out contracting arrangements with the then newly introduced fundholding General Practitioners. With the passage of time, however, this new breed of professional began to share their experiences, and their job became more clearly defined, with the emergence of a set of discrete functions.

Amongst the newly appointed Medical Directors, who on the whole were somewhat bewildered by their new positions, a group of individuals emerged who had a much clearer vision of what the role could and should be. By 1993/1994, the doctors in this group were tackling the Medical Director's remit pro-actively and were determined to play a major role in the strategic direction of their Trusts. They set about developing clear managerial relationships, both with the Chief Executive and with clinical directors. This group of individuals had been meeting under the auspices of the Medical Directors Group of the British Association of Medical Managers (BAMM) and formed the Association of Trust Medical Directors (ATMD) in April 1994, which sits within the BAMM organisation.

By the summer of 1996, the ATMD was in a position to produce a document entitled *Roles and Responsibilities of the Medical Director*,[2] based on an extensive survey of UK Medical Directors, which drew together the key common elements of the job. The circulation of this document also served to enlighten the NHS as to quite how broad and demanding the role of the Medical Director had become. On the other hand, it clearly also engendered some considerable anxiety in those Trusts where the Medical Director was not taking on these duties or was trying to deliver the role with inadequate time, resources or skill.

Alongside the production of this document, Medical Directors had been developing their skills and knowledge at an impressive pace. Many had undertaken some form of management development; others had gained their skills by hard-earned experience. By the time *Roles and Responsibilities*[2] was published, a major change had taken place. Medical Directors were beginning to emerge as key strategic players in Trusts and it was agreed generally that the job simply could not be done on much less than a half-time commitment. Also, there was a distinct change in the type of person appointed to the post. Initially, the role seemed to be the domain of the pre-retirement consultant, the elder statesman, and the well-respected clinician approaching the end of his or her career. These individuals often were expected not to rock the boat, to keep things on an even keel; and they had largely acquired their positions by means of a tap on the shoulder from the Chief Executive, or, as many described it, 'by not jumping back quickly enough when the Chief Executive was looking for volunteers'.

The newer breed of Medical Directors was most certainly younger. They also saw the opportunity as a strategic career step, as a chance to spread wings, broaden horizons and gain valuable experience. Many of this new breed had previously been involved in some form of management development, either through involvement in management projects or as a result of a personal commitment to understanding more about the organisation and how it works. The new breed took the role very seriously, despite the fact that the drawbacks – the constant battle between managerial and clinical demands, the lack of any career progression for those taking on these roles, and a lack of a reward system that would make the post attractive – were, by now, appreciated only too clearly. These issues were fully recognised at this stage as being critical if the role were to attract the brightest and best clinicians.

That said, doctors were – and remain – increasingly attracted to take on the job. Why should this be so? Given the ever-increasing pressure and need to get the quality of clinical care right, the stress of balancing a clinical and a managerial career, with less than excellent rewards, why, then, should doctors take on these posts?

The answer lies in the satisfaction clinicians find in using the insight and skill gained over years and years of operational clinical practice, to improve services for patients. Many doctors have been utterly frustrated for years by working in a system that simply does not support the delivery of excellent health care to patients. This does not, on any account, reflect ill-will or idleness on anyone's part, but is the inevitable consequence of a structure in which those making the policy and managerial decisions do not have the insight and knowledge of those working at the coal face on a day to day basis. Many Medical Directors have commented that, although they may earn less and have much more in the way of hassle, they nevertheless prefer to work in medical management than in a traditional clinical job. It is both intellectually demanding and constantly changing. The ever-present need to develop a creative solution to complex and high-level problems provides a major challenge to doctors' ingenuity and imagination. Many Medical Directors describe a huge sense of achievement when the apparently impossible is made to happen through smart thinking, effective persuasion and leadership. This they describe as by far the most satisfying part of the job.

The past ten years have seen a major change in attitude on the part of medical professionals, from one in which management was a 'dirty word', its sole purpose being to thwart the efforts of clinical professionals, to one in which every doctor has management as part of his or her job, and the choice is whether or not to do that part well and with the appropriate knowledge and skill. These changes, however, have not taken place at the same pace everywhere, nor has the environment of the NHS remained stable.

Today's medical management environment

The past few years have seen major changes in the public's perception, and indeed expectations, of healthcare. In the past, the public had been happy to believe that 'doctor knows best' and was comfortable in accepting the doctor's superior knowledge base. The public also was largely unaware of the major differences in either quality of, or access to, healthcare.

The rate of technological advance has been dramatic over the past decade and has radically altered what can be provided – and therefore what can be demanded and expected of the NHS. Alongside this, exposure on television documentaries of numerous service failures and the frank depiction of the medical world in television drama, 'soaps' and other media forms, all have contributed to a growing public awareness that doctors are indeed fallible human beings. Uncomfortable as this notion might be, the public has realised that healthcare standards in all parts of the country are by no means identical. The ease of access to resources of medical knowledge through the Internet has further empowered members of the public, who are not only becoming aware of the possibilities that healthcare could deliver, but also are far less accepting of the concept of clinical freedom. All of this has led to a turbulent, dynamic environment, further fuelled by a number of very public failures in the systems safeguarding the clinical probity of NHS organisations.

The Bristol heart surgery case in 1998, in which paediatric cardiac surgeons continued to operate despite clear evidence that they should no longer do so, given the mortality of the procedures in their hands, is, perhaps, the most prominent of these failures. This case – along with the failures of cancer screening services, which hit the headlines throughout 1998 – has served as a major catalyst to the current thinking on clinical governance. Indeed, performance of clinical practitioners, along with a growing preoccupation with quality management systems and the added impetus of the failure, formed the core of the quality management aspects of the government's white paper of December 1997, *The New NHS. Modern. Dependable.*[3]

The National Plan for the NHS,[4] launched in July 2000, has taken the quality of clinical care to new levels of scrutiny and action, and redefines the role of the Medical Director in today's NHS. It is a fascinating and demanding role, which should not, on any account, be taken lightly. Above all, the role of Medical Director should not be undertaken by individuals without the appropriate aptitude, knowledge and skills. It is essential that the Trust board ensures that the right individual with the right support, training, development and resources is appointed to this role, which is so critical to the Trust's future health.

The government has taken the concepts of quality management outlined in *A First Class Service. Quality in the New NHS*[5] and developed them into the National Plan, and has set out its determination not only to improve clinical quality, but also to ensure that variation in care standards is removed. The announcement of the major injection of funding into the service in March 2000 galvanised the creation of a series of teams, largely service-based, together forming the Modernisation Action Team (MAT). The five teams represented:

▶ Patient access

▶ Performance and productivity

▶ Partnership

▶ Professional and the workforce

▶ Prevention.

Each team was given the challenge of tackling the implementation of the various strands of the agenda. The fundamental philosophy was that the quality of clinical care and the positioning of the patient must be right in the very centre of thinking and of service design, and that this is no longer an optional extra. The MATs, and the process that surrounded them, for the first time explicitly aligned policy-makers with practitioners, many of whom were medical and nursing leaders, at Trust and Primary Care Group level.

The National Plan for the NHS is based fundamentally on changes in attitude and approach of the professions – to patients and to each other. The way forward for the NHS is one in which revalidation of clinical staff is the norm, and fundamental to this is the process of appraisal – the core of medical management. The Medical Director's role must embrace the implementation of an appraisal system throughout the organisation. The information gained from an appraisal then will feed the revalidation process on an individual basis and the clinical governance process on an aggregate basis.

The practical challenge of managing clinical performance was recognised early on by medical and clinical directors and by the Department of Health. The need to avoid lengthy periods of suspension and to put in place mechanisms to evaluate a clinician's performance was addressed in a document from the Chief Medical Officer, Professor Liam Donaldson, in December 1999. The document, *Supporting Doctors, Protecting Patients*,[6] outlines a range of assessment services and mechanisms. These will ensure that doctors who are felt to be performing less than optimally, for whatever reason, will be identified early and assessed for their clinical and behavioural competence. Following the assessment process, a series of recommendations will be made to the Trust in terms of action for the individual.

Clinical governance and the Medical Director

In the pursuit of effective clinical governance, the Medical Director and his or her counterpart in nursing management are the key players. The case study described below outlines some of the issues involved.

The first duty of any Medical Director in delivering clinical governance must be to ensure that systems to pick up quality failures are in place. It is all too easy, however, to make the assumption that once the basic systems are in place, no more need be done, the box is checked and everyone can relax.

It is crucial that the temptation to blindly set up systems, technology and committee structures as the 'answer' to clinical governance is firmly resisted.

It is fundamental to understand that the key to managing clinical performance – and to achieving clinical governance – is mastering the art of influencing colleagues, the peers with whom the individual has – in all probability – worked for many years. The Medical Director must persuade them, at the very minimum, that if their clinical performance is not of an acceptable standard, it will simply not be tolerated. Clinical governance means creating an environment in which all clinical professionals are motivated and inspired to improve their clinical and professional performance, even

---

Box 6.1. A case study: The issues

Dr Wellman, Medical Director at Heartwood Hospital, was having a trying day. The chief cause of his concern was Andrew Thompson, the senior surgeon in the hospital. Although Andrew had no formal managerial role in the Trust, he was nevertheless extremely influential as the 'elder statesman' surgeon. Gordon Wellman had become increasingly concerned about the infection rate from Andrew's team, particularly in his cholecystectomy patients. An audit had been undertaken 18 months previously and the audit team had felt that, as a whole, the surgical infection rates were high. The Directorate Team had drawn up a set of guidelines, and all the surgeons had agreed to change their practice. Now, 18 months on, although the infection rate across the directorate had improved, Andrew's rates were as high, if not higher than they were before.

Gordon had been acutely embarrassed by a conversation with Becky Morris, Nurse Manager in the Surgical Directorate. Becky had been concerned for some time about Mr Thompson's behaviour in theatre. He was rude and aggressive on many occasions and frequently late for lists. Furthermore, as she observed tartly, 'It's a waste of time drawing up guidelines – the good ones take them on board anyway, but Andrew won't listen to anyone but himself. He always does his own thing.'

Four miles across the city, at the Royal Hospital, Dr John Burton, Medical Director, was frowning over the list of consultants applying for management training courses. He had masterminded the implementation of an appraisal system for all consultant staff two years previously. The initial first year had been extremely hard work, not only in terms of getting through the appraisal session with each of the 108 consultants, and the subsequent follow-up personal-development meetings, but also in terms of training the clinical directors in conducting the appraisals themselves. This year, however, the process had been somewhat less stressful with the clinical directors taking on much more of the load.

Dr Burton is keen to be as accommodating as possible to the consultants. However, each consultant has his or her clinical continuing medical education (CME) accredits to achieve, and time and resources are limited. The dilemma John Burton now faces is how to allocate the meagre management development budget fairly amongst the consultant staff, whilst at the same time ensuring that the skills and knowledge most needed by the Trust broadly matches those of the individuals. 'I have to say that what I think is needed and what they think they need are sometimes entirely different things,' he mused, 'but I'm still really pleased that the colleagues are showing such enthusiasm.'

The management philosophy at the Royal, developed over the past five years between John Burton and Mark Winston, Chief Executive, was one of ensuring that effective systems are in place to monitor the quality of clinical practice. Thus, clinical audit, risk management, patient feedback, outcome measures and process improvement systems had been developed over the years in a structured programme, alongside an active approach to developing strong clinical leadership. These systems, however, are only ever as good as the individuals concerned, and the ability of these individuals to influence their clinical colleagues. The Trust's executive team, having placed considerable emphasis on the systems development side over the past five years, is now fairly confident that quality failures will be picked up swiftly. The predominant emphasis now at the Royal is on developing individuals and encouraging them to adopt a more proactive approach – preventing disasters before they have a chance to happen.

---

though it may already be of a high standard. Clearly, the challenges that face the Medical Director vary greatly, depending on the nature of the Trust and the type of management systems that are in place to monitor quality.

This fundamental management challenge – developing the right culture to allow quality improvement to take place – is common to every Trust and Primary Care

Organisation. The fact that has to be faced is that no one can change an individual's clinical practice other than the individual him/herself. Information can be produced, mission statements can be issued, policies and guidelines can be circulated, persuasion, exhortation and peer pressure can be brought to bear – but unless the clinician has made a conscious decision to change or improve the way he or she performs, nothing will happen. Changing clinical behaviour is notoriously difficult. As the nurse manager in the case described above quite rightly observed, the 'good', conscientious clinicians, who are by far in the majority, are keen to improve their practice anyway; after all, no clinician sets off to do the job poorly in the first place. However, there are a small number of doctors who are simply unwilling to change their practice and indeed do not see any need to do so.

Clinical governance aims to develop and enhance clinical practice amongst the good, whilst simultaneously providing a set of systems to ensure that poor practice is identified, the lessons learnt implemented into clinical practice and the effect of these lessons monitored.

The two Trusts described in the case have very different approaches and have very different perspectives on the introduction of clinical governance. However, the huge difference between the organisations is only really appreciated by the small number of clinical staff who hold sessions in both Trusts.

The nuts and bolts of clinical governance must be in place at directorate or service level. The Medical Director cannot and should not personally oversee every consultant or process. With the development of clinical governance, the Medical Director's role

---

Box 6.2. Three months later

Back at Heartwood hospital, things are not going at all well. Andrew Thompson lost his temper with a senior theatre nurse last week, swore at her and was both threatening and abusive to her. The scene was witnessed by Dr Malcolm Neil, a newly appointed consultant anaesthetist. Dr Neil mainly works at the Royal but also covers two lists each week at Heartwood and had recently taken on Andrew Thompson's list. Dr Neil is hoping to take over as clinical director of anaesthesia at the Royal and has a keen interest in quality management models.

'I am just appalled by this man's behaviour,' he mused to himself, 'but what's the right thing to do? The management lot at Heartwood don't seem to be interested and yet this man is going to do some real damage before too long – if he's not already done so. We have ways of picking all this up at the Royal, but nothing here at Heartwood so I'm now left with the question of whether I should report him. If I do, it's not going to win me any friends – but if I don't, maybe *I'm* in the wrong. I'm sure the latest guidance from the GMC makes that clear.' Finally, Dr Neil decides to have an informal word with John Burton at the Royal, who, whilst busy, as always, is happy to spend half an hour chatting about the matter.

Meanwhile at Heartwood, Gordon Wellman had just received a formal complaint about Andrew Thompson from Becky Morris. He was at his desk, considering what to do, when the telephone rang. 'The Chairman and I wondered if you could pop over for a few minutes?' the Trust's Chief Executive Paul Johnson said, 'We've got some pretty serious complaints we need to discuss with you.' Dr Wellman made his way over to the executive offices with a heavy heart.

Over at the Royal, Dr Neil was feeling somewhat more optimistic. He had had the chance to talk things through with John Burton and had decided to confront both Gordon Wellman and Paul Johnson at Heartwood the next day.

becomes quite clear. As the guardian of clinical probity, the Medical Director must be confident that effective systems and effective clinical leadership are in place for each and every clinical service within the Trust. That said, the Medical Director also must know how to deal effectively, appropriately and skilfully with any clinician whose performance is falling below the expected standard.

This is often a complex business, with multiple aspects. The colleague may be ill, stressed, or behaving in an unacceptable manner, or they may be incompetent. However, most problems with colleagues do not present with a single convenient label on them. Most are multifaceted, with information presenting from every direction at random. The Medical Director must constantly be on the alert for patterns of unusual behaviour amongst clinical colleagues. The Medical Director must be close enough to the action to know when things are going wrong and to be closely connected to the internal, informal networks of the Trust. At the same time, however, he or she also must stand back sufficiently to view the organisation as a whole and set the issues within the right context.

It is the Medical Director's responsibility to make sure that the culture and environment is one in which poor performance and clinical risk are managed with skill and sensitivity. Consultants, and particularly clinical directors, must be made fully aware of how much of the monitoring and indeed investigation of questionable performance should be undertaken and at what stage the matter should be reported to the Medical Director. There must, of course, be a full and open relationship between the Medical Director, clinical director and consultant colleagues. Without this, the Medical Director cannot hope to be successful in clinical governance.

Consider the Trusts outlined in the case. At the Royal, considerable effort has been put into developing a system. The philosophy of the Trust is clearly articulated, at every step of the management process. The process, which provides a useful vehicle for discussing performance and the needs for further professional development, also provides a mechanism for managing staff morale and health. An important byproduct, however, is the opportunity the process provides to develop the informal network, to gain the soft information of who is doing what, and which areas of the Trust the Medical Director might wish to focus on most clearly.

The appraisal process makes staff feel valued. It is sobering to reflect on the lack of attention that has been paid to the individual clinician's satisfaction with his or her job or career. As one consultant remarked, rather sadly, 'This is the first time in 30 years anyone has ever asked or cared about what I do next.'

In contrast, at Heartwood, each and every problem in the service will come as an unpleasant surprise, simply because the ethos of pro-actively seeking out the problems is not there, and Gordon Wellman does not have the 'inside knowledge' he needs to be effective. The Trust management is therefore set on the back foot and is constantly reacting to issues that could and should have been prevented.

There are many, varied calls upon the Medical Director's time. As most Medical Directors are still working clinically, time is indeed under pressure. However, of all the many things a Medical Director must do, this determination to create the right culture and the right networks is top priority. Without it, the role as a Medical Director is totally reactive and as such is not really manageable. At the Royal, John Burton has created a culture that will support him in his job, and has put an appraisal system in place. There are, in fact, many other ways of changing the culture of an organisation and the true art is in identifying the mechanism most likely to bring about change, given the nature of the Trust.

Box 6.3. The next day

Malcolm Neil arrived early for his list at Heartwood Hospital. He had arranged to have a word with Gordon Wellman and Paul Johnson before he went to theatre, although now he was beginning to question the wisdom of his actions. His confidence of the previous evening had evaporated on his arrival at Heartwood, and now he desperately wished he'd kept quiet. As he began to explain his concerns to the Medical Director and Chief Executive, he sensed that Gordon Wellman was already somewhat stressed and irritated at his remarks. Paul Johnson, on the other hand, listened calmly and encouraged Malcolm to expand on his anxieties about Andrew Thompson's performance. 'It's no use avoiding the issue any more. Something's just got to be done!' Gordon Wellman was almost shouting. 'Why is this sort of thing always happening here? Can't we have some sort of quality policy in this place to stop all this nonsense?' Malcolm Neil was not terribly sure what to say about all this but began, anyway, to describe some of the processes in place at the Royal. Again, Paul Johnson listened carefully, and Malcolm left for his list feeling that at least no harm had been done.

Two days later, John Burton at the Royal was slightly surprised to hear from Paul Johnson at Heartwood. Paul had spoken to Mark Winston and had asked if both Chief Executives and Medical Directors could get together one evening for a drink to explore the possibility of sharing the Royal's approach to performance management with colleagues at Heartwood.

It is not easy to be a Medical Director. In many ways, clinical governance has clarified the issues, but at the same time has given the role considerable breadth and complexity, along with accountability for the fundamental priority in healthcare – the quality of clinical practice. It is therefore absolutely essential that Medical Directors do the job well – a poorly performing Medical Director does no one any service and can cause considerable damage (see Box 6.4).

What makes a good Medical Director?

First and foremost must come judgement. Just as in the clinical world, the facts and figures may be there, the whys and wherefores evident. The real skill, however, lies in the Medical Director's judgement, timing, sensitivity and knowledge of how both the individuals and the organisation itself will react – and his/her ability to use this skill to make things happen.

Second, there is a menu of skills without which the Medical Director simply cannot survive. In terms of the clinical governance agenda, these must include risk and crisis management, and dealing with the poorly performing colleagues. Medical Directors also must know enough about the systems that should be in place to spot when they are not functioning properly. Medical Directors must, above all, know when the limits of their own knowledge have been reached – and they certainly must not be too proud to ask for help when they know they are in trouble. Finally – and perhaps this should come first – Medical Directors should know how to communicate effectively, not only with patients but also with colleagues, at board level, with the public, with the other clinical disciplines and with the media. All the knowledge and skill is useless if the ideas are not communicated effectively. If the key to buying a new business property is *location, location, location*, the key to effective medical directoring must be *communicate, communicate, communicate*.

All this may seem a daunting prospect; and yet, the real opportunity afforded by clinical governance and The National Plan cannot be ignored by Medical Directors. Clinical governance provides not only a framework for the task of the Medical Director, but also provides the legitimacy and the power to demand demonstrable standards of quality in clinical care. For years, clinicians – even those in medical management positions – have struggled with improving service quality, without the benefit of a nationally driven framework. Clinical governance, now sitting within the National Plan for the NHS, provides that framework. It is time for clinicians, and medical managers in particular, to demonstrate their determination to ensure clinical governance makes a real difference to the quality of care the NHS provides.

Box 6.4. Clinical governance and the Medical Director

▶ Clinical governance happens at directorate or service level; the Medical Director's job is to create the right environment to liberate and empower Clinical Directors to deliver clinical governance, through leadership and management systems.

▶ The Medical Director, along with management and clinical colleagues, should regard the development of a pro-active, energetic approach to managing the quality of clinical performance as his or her topmost priority.

▶ The Medical Director must take every step to ensure that each clinical service or specialty has effective and efficient clinical leadership, and has high-quality management and information systems.

▶ The Medical Director must be able to demonstrate with confidence, that for each service or specialty, the quality of clinical care is monitored, and, when lacking, that lessons are learnt and implemented.

▶ The Medical Director must develop robusts informal networks with the Clinical Directors, other clinicians and managers, which will allow a detailed knowledge and 'feel' for the organisation whilst simultaneously keeping an organisation-wide perspective.

▶ Communication, time management, investigation and influencing skills are key requirements.

References

1   Department of Health. *Working for Patients*. London: The Stationery Office, 1991.
2   Association of Trust Medical Directors. *Roles and Responsibilities of the Medical Director*, 1996; ISBN 1 900120 02X.
3   Department of Health. *The New NHS. Modern. Dependable*. Command paper 3807. London, December 1997.
4   Secretary of State for Health. *The NHS Plan. Plan for Investment, a Plan for Reform*. London: The Stationery Office, 2000.
5   Department of Health. *A First Class Service. Quality in the New NHS*. Wetherby: Department of Health. 1998.
6   Department of Health. *Supporting Doctors, Protecting Patients*. London: The Stationery Office, 1999.

7

Learning From Complaints

Susan Hobbs

Introduction

In general terms, most patients, their families, friends and carers have considerable trust in the services that the NHS provides. The majority of patients experience high-quality care but where they perceive a drop in standards they have a right to be heard and for their complaints to be dealt with promptly, efficiently and politely.

So why do people complain about the health service? It is widely accepted that the NHS is an incredibly complex organisation. In total, it employs over one million staff. It treats more and more people year on year, providing more and more complex care, pushing back the very frontiers of science and technology, yet many consumers of a service that is considered internationally by many as the epitome of good practice remain dissatisfied. Arguably, the very nature and complexity of such a service would suggest that it was never – or never will be – a perfect service; so what has changed recently to develop a more consumer focus on the delivery of health services?

In the past 20 years, the public sector in virtually all industrialised nations has changed dramatically. Long-held assumptions about the role and function of the public sector have been removed, to be replaced by ideas largely borrowed from private sector business and performance measures, strategic and business planning, the importance of management information, increased accountability and the pressures of the internal market. Add to that shift the continuous and very public pattern and pace of change, which has set the agenda for the NHS since the 1990 reforms. In particular, there has been the introduction of the Patients' Charter, the very essence of which was to widen choice and to make the health service more responsive to patients' needs. All have further raised public expectations of a service that is arguably unable to meet the level of quality to which it aspires. The public and media interest in all things clinical, whether fact or fiction – and sometimes it is difficult to tell the difference – have all changed our overall perceptions of the health service. Indeed, the consumer's expectations of the public sector, fuelled for some by increasing wealth and for others – the old, the sick and the poor – by increasing needs, continue to rise and be disappointed.

What triggers complaints?

We know that people complain for different reasons. The Wilson report[1] stressed that all complainants want to be taken seriously. The committee commented that:

Complainants can face an uphill struggle when using the NHS Complaints Procedures, firstly in making their views known and secondly in receiving the sort of response they would wish for.

There is no doubt that complainants want their views to be acknowledged. They want an explanation, and they also want the individual or the organisation they hold responsible to be prepared to take action and to be told what has been done to put matters right. To maintain public confidence in the NHS, it is essential that all complaints be investigated thoroughly and without bias.

Complainants, particularly if they are patients, often feel uneasy about voicing their concerns in the first place. Many genuinely feel that by complaining about any aspect of treatment and care they are jeopardising any further treatment that may be required. They usually are not in a powerful position; they feel vulnerable; and the ability of the organisation to respond positively and quickly will become the benchmark for the resolution of the issue. Others often feel that the whole process is an exercise in damage limitation.

A simple apology may be what the complainant really wants. The apology should be unconditional; if this is not forthcoming, the complainant is less likely to be satisfied. Experience tells us that all too often a failure or unwillingness to apologise at an early stage is the reason for complaints proceeding further through the system than is really necessary or appropriate. Recent research found that most complainants only wanted an apology and to be convinced that the same thing would not happen to others.

One particular report[2] stated that in 70% of incidents progress to litigation would not have happened if there were an early apology. It would appear that it is better to seek out possible dissatisfactions than let the situation escalate to anger or a formal complaint, which puts staff on the defensive, initiates worries about legal liability if a mistake is admitted and draws the battle lines. Many complaints' officers and others who investigate complaints are fearful of the risk of litigation. If this is a real possibility, a clear policy must be agreed which allows clinical and managerial staff to give full and honest explanations to patients and relatives on humanitarian and clinical grounds, even at the risk of ensuing litigation. When something has gone wrong, taking an active stance in communicating with patients and carers so that early restorative action can be initiated before they complain can only be beneficial. As many patients sue partly because they want an explanation,[3,4] this is probably a sound financial policy as well as a humane one.

Equally, some complainants also may want action that has a more direct bearing on the nature of the care provided to them, such as faster or additional treatment, or financial compensation. However, even in cases relating to clinical judgement, complainants do not always have financial compensation as a primary goal. Some who go on to take legal action do so simply because other goals are not being met.

Sadly, complaints about the NHS are viewed by some staff as an irritating intrusion; some colleagues are often immediately defensive and resistant to any investigation taking place into their own clinical practice, even to the point of obstruction.

Changing policies

Reference was made earlier to the Wilson report.[1] This came about as a result of a thorough and far-reaching review of complaints procedures that the government of the day announced in 1993 in response to mounting criticism of the previous complaints procedure. The shortcomings of the previous system were widely described as follows:

▶ Complainants faced an uphill struggle to make their views known and in receiving the sort of response they would wish for.

▶ People did not know who to complain to.

▶ Too many different procedures and people were involved.

▶ NHS procedures were seen often to be ineffective in meeting complainants objectives and would often increase dissatisfaction.

▶ Very few organisations had any visible written information about the complaints system.

To address these issues, a committee, chaired by Professor Alan Wilson, Vice Chancellor of Leeds University, was established by the then Secretary of State. Its objective was to review the procedures available for making and handling complaints by NHS patients and their families in the United Kingdom and the costs and benefits of finding alternatives to current procedures. The committee reviewed practice in the NHS, as well as examples of different approaches in both the public and private sectors in Britain and in the health service of other countries. The committee recommended that the following principles should be incorporated into NHS complaints procedures:

▶ Responsiveness

▶ Quality enhancement

▶ Cost-effectiveness

▶ Accessibility

▶ Impartiality

▶ Simplicity

▶ Speed

▶ Confidentiality

▶ Accountability.

A report, published by the committee in May 1994, recommended major changes based on three principles:

▶ There should be a common system for complaints covering all NHS services.

▶ The system should be geared to the complainants concerns and disciplinary action should be kept separate.

▶ There should be a two-stage approach: the first inhouse, starting where the complaint arises; the second an investigation by an independent panel.

Full guidance on the implementation of the agreed new NHS Complaints Procedure was introduced in March 1996,[5] and NHS Trusts, Health Authorities, Family Health Service Authorities and GPs were expected to design and operate their own complaints procedures, using the guidance document as a framework, while adhering to the legal requirements of the appropriate directions and regulations.

The key objectives for the new procedure reinforced the guiding principles, and all NHS organisations were expected to demonstrate and reinforce compliance. The monitoring of complaints procedures, and in particular the attainment of compliance to targets, has become part of the contract monitoring arrangements. From a commissioning perspective, and in the absence of formal accreditation systems, new complaints procedures should be seen enforceable through contracting mechanisms as part of quality monitoring.

Effective complaints management

The effective management of complaints should be of prime importance to any organisation committed to improving service quality. The manner in which a complaint is received, and the speed and sincerity with which issues are addressed, contribute to the perception of the organisation by users of its services, members of staff and the wider community. However, given that the number of complaints grow year on year, the complexity increases and many complainants remain dissatisfied long after the final letter is signed, we may well not have got it quite right yet. Major organisational changes such as NHS Trust reconfigurations, the development of Local Health Groups (Wales) and Primary Care Groups/Trusts (England) present a perfect opportunity to review and improve complaints management. In addition, the baseline assessments which all NHS organisations undertook in 1999, as part of the introduction of clinical governance, raised issues relating to several components of the current policy. Also, there is currently a national review of complaints management in process, commissioned by the Department of Health, which will be completed in December 2000. This review concentrates on the complaints process itself as well as the experiences of users and managers. An interim report from this review highlights several key areas for improvement:

▶ Ease of access and ease of use for complainants.

▶ Improved training for complaints managers.

▶ Local resolution to remain the primary objective.

▶ Consistency of approach.

▶ Clear process for dealing with multi-agency complaints.

▶ Better feedback for complainants and staff.

▶ Learning from complaints.

▶ Sharing best practice.

▶ Educating the public and their advocates.

Customer care training

During the past ten years, much emphasis has been placed upon enabling staff to respond positively to patients' and carers' concerns, questions and criticisms, and to improve information. The use of the word 'customer' was anathema in the public sector and any discussion about how staff possibly could be trained to respond better to patients largely fell on deaf ears. Indeed, a huge and challenging cultural shift has had to be effected in many NHS organisations for customer care training to be accepted as an essential component of the education and training portfolio. Learning how to handle and diffuse difficult situations, including managing potential complainants, is an integral part of customer care training and arguably should be mandatory for every new member of staff who has a role which brings him or her into direct contact with patients and carers.

In addition, there should be specific training for a wide range of staff in dealing with dissatisfied customers. This training should be considered to be as important as any other, and as such should be planned and funded as part of the organisational development and training programme. Locally, following a survey of medical students, a one-day programme has been developed jointly between the Trust and the College of Medicine. The programme covers many aspects of risk management, including scenario planning and the handling of complaints. Non-attendance is not an option. It is clear, from regularly reviewing complaints, that we certainly need to accept that empathy, sympathy and the ability to admit mistakes are attributes that many clinical and managerial colleagues need to acquire and maintain. Support, and even counselling, for colleagues involved directly in disturbing or injurious incidents also should be available if considered appropriate.

Guiding principles

Complaints should not be seen as the sole responsibility of a corporate department. With an increasing emphasis on personal accountability, everyone in the organisation needs to contribute to:

▶ handling them effectively

▶ improving performance in complaints management, and

▶ learning the lessons from them.

Handling complaints properly is an important part of good customer care. It shows that you:

▶ listen to your users views

▶ learn from your mistakes, and

▶ are continually trying to improve your service.

Ensuring access to the Complaints Procedure is simple and understood; it will:

▶ encourage complaints and compliments by advertising your procedures and making them easy to use

▶ inform all your users about your service standards and how to comment if you do not meet them

▶ make it clear to the public that you welcome complaints and comments and that you will use the information to improve your services

▶ make you think about providing a service for users who have special needs, for example those with a reading, hearing or language difficulty, and

▶ enable you to regularly audit your procedures.

A good idea is to enhance support for staff by putting together 'survival' kits on handling complaints at ward/departmental level. This will:

▶ encourage frontline staff to 'own' complaints

▶ give staff immediate access to clear written procedures that focus on sorting out complaints quickly, and

▶ provide immediate support for staff – in particular new or locum staff.

But one must remember the following:

▶ Consult staff and users when drawing up and revising complaints procedures.

▶ Make sure that the procedures are fair to staff and users, and that information is treated as confidential.

▶ Recognise the importance of good communication skills when recruiting and training staff who handle complaints.

▶ Make sure that all staff know about the policy and receive training.

▶ Draw up a menu of remedies and make sure that staff and users understand the options, including the role of the Ombudsman.

▶ Support your staff, which, in turn, will improve their commitment to handling complaints properly.

▶ Get the basics right: listen carefully and investigate properly.

Complaints and performance management

▶ Record all complaints and analyse them regularly to understand users' views and the improvements they want to see.

▶ Establish an effective complaints monitoring group, preferably with membership from the Community Health Council, or other patients representatives.

▶ Collate regular reports to management teams, looking at trends and changes in the pattern of complaints which may arise as a result of changes in service delivery or configuration.

▶ Report formally at least quarterly to the board.

▶ Publish information in the Annual Report, or equivalent, on:

    ▶ trends

    ▶ issues for complaints management, and

    ▶ lessons learned.

▶ Pass information from complaints monitoring to policy makers.

▶ Take advantage of new information technology.

▶ Subject complaints monitoring to peer review.

Local resolution

The local resolution stage provides the quickest and fullest opportunity for investigation and resolution of the complaint. The aim is to satisfy the complainant while at the same time being fair to staff. This process must be fair, open, flexible and conciliatory to both staff and complainants. The Department of Health places great emphasis on resolving complaints as quickly as possible. It is a mandatory process and therefore a comprehensive entity in its own right, and not simply a run up to an independent review. The Medical Defence Union (MDU) also supports strongly the principle of local resolution of complaints. Anecdotal evidence suggests that properly handled local procedures will resolve around 75% of grievances. Speed, sympathy and a willingness to listen may be all that is necessary.

Independent review

Complainants who remain dissatisfied at the end of the local resolution process may refer a request for an independent review to the Trust or Health Authority convenor either orally or in writing. The complainant has 20 days in which to lodge this appeal. Requests for independent review are considered by a Convenor, usually a non-executive director of a NHS Trust or Health Authority whose role is a vital part of the process. Training for these individuals is essential, as is having the right background, experience and personal qualities. The prime function of the Convenor is to consider the complainant's request for an independent review of their case where it has not been possible to resolve the matter locally. He/she will also sit on the panel if one is convened. From the statement or letter from the complainant, the convenor will wish to assess whether or not there is a further case to answer. Many complaints that arrive at this stage usually describe a major dissatisfaction with the process itself, as well as the described inadequacies or poor outcome of treatment and care. Often they arise from highly complex cases where many clinicians have been involved and stark inconsistencies appear.

The importance at the local resolution stage of a senior and responsible manager investigating thoroughly before pulling together the final reply cannot be overstated. This is essential to ensure that there is consistency of approach and that the response is factually accurate and all those involved can feel ownership of the issues, long before the Chief Executive signs the final response.

In making the decision to set up a panel, the Convenor will consult with an independent lay-chairman appointed from the regional list and also will take appropriate and independent clinical advice. The final decision, however, rests with the Convenor.

In summary, the Convenor's role is to:

▶ ensure impartiality

▶ ascertain whether all the opportunities for satisfying the complainant have been exhausted

▶ determine whether or not a panel might be able to resolve the complaint

▶ agree terms of reference, and

▶ report his/her decision to the complainant and to the Trust or Health Authority.

Health Service Commissioner (the Ombudsman)

All complainants have the option at any stage of the process to refer their complaint to the Ombudsman, who has jurisdiction over the whole range of NHS complaints, except personnel or contractual complaints. He/she has complete discretion as to when to start an investigation, or when to stop it; the only time when he/she may hesitate is if there is also a claim for negligence under investigation. The Ombudsman's investigations are thorough, and he/she has the power of the High Court to compel managers to produce documents, and to provide witnesses for interview. Whilst he/she has no mandatory or executive power by which to compel an organisation to change anything, a Trust or Health Authority could find themselves in the annual report and/or the subject of a parliamentary select committee. In short, doing nothing is not really an option.

Complaints and risk management

No organisation can devote sufficient resources to eliminate all risks; things will inevitably go wrong. Just as aircraft will crash, banks will be defrauded and oil tankers will sink, healthcare professionals will give incorrect treatment or a lack of care.

Risk management is an organisational response to a need to reduce errors and their costs. In most NHS Trusts, risk management is now regarded as an integral component of the general management process, not an optional extra. It has clear links with quality improvement programmes; but more than with other quality assurance initiatives, it places a special emphasis on the costs and consequences of poor-quality care. Risk management is fundamentally a particular approach to improving the quality of care, which places particular emphasis on occasions in which patients are harmed or disturbed by their treatment or care. Thus, a coherent, comprehensive and accessible complaints management policy should be accepted as an essential component of the overall risk management strategy. The prompt management of complaints, avoidance of litigation or the early settlement of damages should benefit both the complainant and Trusts.

The interplay of human and organisational factors that result in errors is complex.[6] Adverse occurrences in patient care are not uncommon,[7] and although only a small proportion of these result in significant damage or distress and even fewer in litigation, much unnecessary distress arises from failure to deal honestly and effectively with such events as they occur. Often, patients are denied what they need most – an explanation of what happened – and when this fails to materialise, they are forced into lodging a formal complaint.

The complaints procedure may be protracted, even when it does not proceed beyond the local system. The cost of dealing with even minor deficiencies in care, in terms of patient or carer distress, can escalate wildly. Dealing promptly and effectively with complaints is part of risk management. To do this, an open approach to complaints management and their antecedents – adverse events and mishaps – is needed.

Case studies

It is always valuable to look at other organisations' case histories; sometimes when reading them, it seems that they must be fictional. In fact, the following are all taken from one Trust complaints tracking system during one year. The names used are fictitious, but the issues identified and the actions taken as a result are real. All make salutary reading.

Case 1

Mrs B, a 69-year-old lady, was admitted to hospital in January 1999. She was assessed in the admissions unit and then transferred to a medical ward. She was seen and examined by a number of medical staff and a provisional diagnosis of a chest infection was made; she also was described in the nursing notes as being anxious. The following day, she was transferred to a gynaecology ward; treatment was instigated and she also received oxygen therapy. Mrs B presumably had been transferred to the gynaecology ward because of a shortage of medical beds, but no one told her or her family why. The nursing and medical notes were both poor. Two days later, the nursing notes indicated that she had felt nauseous and had subsequently vomited. It also was noted that she had slept poorly and complained of sweating. Twelve hours later, however, it was recorded that she was feeling brighter; no entry was made between times.

In the early hours of the next day, a note was made to the effect that Mrs B had refused her antibiotics as a result of still feeling nauseous. At this point, she was prescribed and given an anti-emetic; she was still receiving oxygen via a nebuliser. Later that day, she was transferred once again to another, different, medical ward. Her daughter and son were, at this point, told different stories as to the function of the new ward: rehabilitation, acute medicine and infectious diseases. Obviously, this created real concern and confusion for the patient – already anxious – and her family. Given that the family knew that Mrs B had a chest infection, they could not relate this new ward to their mother's needs. The family then became concerned about continuity of care: on the previous ward Mrs B had all of her care needs met by the nursing staff, on this ward, within the same 24-hour period, Mrs B was left to care for herself.

Concern also was raised about Mrs B being allowed to go to the toilet unassisted when quite clearly she could not manage; particularly that she was on a diuretic and there was no fluid balance chart. In addition, there was only one entry in the nursing notes that addressed her mobility needs, which also became a problem for discharge planning. The outcome was a loss of confidence in the nursing team by the family, who considered that either they did not understand her needs or were unaware of her true physical condition, or just did not care about Mrs B.

Issues

▶ Communication

▶ Documentation

▶ Nursing care

▶ Excessive transfers.

Outcome

The complaint was not resolved easily and did go to independent review. One of the recommendations of the Independent Review Panel was that there should be a complete review of nursing records to ensure that detailed account of a patient's history and nursing needs can be identified clearly. The Panel was critical of the nursing notes, which were confusing; there was little evidence of real assessment and no evaluation of the care given.

The Panel also felt that the importance of good communication and early explanation of intentions or changes must be made to patients and their families. Members of the nursing staff interviewed by the Panel appeared reluctant to accept any responsibility for the distress caused to Mrs B and her family. The Panel also was highly critical of three moves in four days.

Finally there was concern expressed that there was a significant loss of confidence in the NHS at a time when the patient had been found to have a chronic illness.

Action taken

This complaint was used as a case study within the directorate. A protocol has been agreed between the medical admissions unit and bed management regarding inappropriate transfer. The skill mix of nurses on the final ward has been reassessed and some grades changed. Workshops on the better use of nursing notes and accountability in practice were used positively. One member of staff has moved on.

Case 2

A young woman was admitted to hospital to deliver a child. The child was born with a deformity to an upper limb, and the family agreed that, as this was a distressing deformity, they did not wish the facts to be made public and that they would tell people in their own time. They were further distressed to learn that at least two of their neighbours knew of the defect within two days of the birth. One neighbour even came to the grandparent's house to offer condolences. At the same time, a relative of the family was employed by the hospital in another clinical area. The family alleged that this person had discovered the information easily and had passed it on to the individuals concerned. It was further complicated by the fact that the complainants felt that the matter had not been dealt with properly and that they had been refused an interview to discuss the matter further. They also wanted disciplinary action taken against the staff member concerned and had great difficulty in separating the two issues. This case remains unresolved as far as the family is concerned, even though it has gone to an Independent Review Panel and was not fully upheld.

Issues

▶ Confidentiality

▶ Abuse of position (staff)

▶ Delays in complaints management system

▶ Access to medical notes.

Action taken

No disciplinary action was taken as a result of the investigation, but all staff have been reminded of their privileged position in relation to confidential and sensitive information. The induction programme for all staff also has been strengthened.

Medical records have reviewed and improved tracer systems for notes, which are no longer left outside the patient's door in the maternity unit. A review of complaints management has been undertaken and the changes implemented as a result, supported by the Trust board.

Case 3

Mrs B was admitted to a district general hospital as an emergency admission with severe airway obstruction, secondary to a large benign goitre. She was known to be asthmatic but had been in reasonable health before this obstruction episode. On admission, her trachea was intubated by an anaesthetist and she was stabilised in the intensive care unit whilst her lungs recovered from the effects of the crisis that had occurred around the admission. She remained intubated until a tracheostomy was performed, and after that a tracheostomy tube (of a Portex type) maintained the patency of her airway. Later, when considered stable, she was transferred to an ENT ward. Despite the Portex tube, her airway became blocked, once again necessitating oro-tracheal intubation. This was converted promptly to tracheal intubation with a special tracheal tube.

Some four weeks after the emergency admission, Mrs B was transferred as an elective transfer to a teaching hospital for further management of her goitre. She was transferred by ambulance to an ENT ward, but was by this time largely self-caring, walking to the ward toilet as required. Tracheostomy care was being provided by the nursing staff with a regimen that included two-hourly suction. Suction was planned for 00:15, but at 23:50 the patient was found to be in respiratory difficulty by a trained nurse. Subsequently, the patient suffered a cardio-respiratory arrest, during which she incurred hypoxic/ischaemic brain damage.

Several issues were raised after the event; these included the integrity of the equipment available, the arrest procedure itself and the training and responsiveness of clinical and administrative staff. There seems little doubt that the incident contributed significantly to Mrs B's death some two months later.

Issues

▶ Safety of the environment on transfer

▶ Resuscitation equipment

▶ Management of emergency

▶ Staff training

▶ Communication.

Action taken

This case was presented to the Risk Management Committee, and key members were asked to discuss the issues and bring back an action plan. Although it was considered that the patient was transferred to a safe environment, it also was considered that the staffing level and skill mix could have been enhanced, even though the patient was essentially self-caring. Cardiac arrest procedures have been reviewed and additional training agreed. Moreover, equipment has been updated and associated training agreed for staff.

Case 4

Mr H, aged 68, was admitted in May 1998 having experienced an episode of throat and chest pain. An electrocardiogram (ECG) was recorded and showed no acute changes, and he was admitted to a medical ward with a diagnosis of acute angina. He was given a bed under the care of a gastroenterologist, who was the physician on take that day. However, the physician was away and the take was being managed by another specialist – not a Cardiologist – who did not at any time see Mr H.

During the night, Mr H experienced periods of pain. This pain was treated by the nursing staff with glyceryl trinitrate (GTN) spray and was recorded in the nursing notes. The next day, Mr H was seen by a senior registrar, the diagnosis was confirmed and a nursing management plan and serial ECGs agreed. These ECGs were taken at 11:00 and were seen by the pre-registration house officer, who interpreted the results and discussed them with his senior house officer. They agreed that, as Mr H was no longer experiencing any pain, he should continue to be cared for under the agreed patient plan. Neither doctor saw or examined Mr H.

Subsequent examination of the relevant ECGs by the Independent Panel's clinical advisers showed that there had been significant changes which indicated a myocardial infarction. Later that morning, the medical notes recorded that he had complained of further chest pains, which were eventually relieved by GTN spray. No entries from the medical team were recorded during the whole of the next day. At 05:00 hours on the following morning, Mr H suffered a further myocardial infarction and died.

In November 1998, his daughter wrote to the Trust complaining of the inadequacy of his medical care. She was particularly concerned that, despite his medical history and the symptoms displayed on admission to hospital, Mr H had not been admitted to a coronary care unit. She also questioned why he had not been admitted under the care of a more appropriate physician and why he had not been prescribed streptokinase. Further correspondence between January and June 1999 restated her complaints; she asked for an Independent Review, and also stressed her view that the two junior doctors had failed to interpret the various ECGs correctly. In the interim, Miss H also had met with the admitting physician and a cardiologist (employed by the Trust) who then proceeded to give his own opinion, which was not necessarily consistent with Trust policy. This complaint went to Independent Review.

Issues

▶ Errors in diagnosis and treatment

▶ Admission policies

▶ Supervision of junior staff

▶ Treatment protocols

▶ Differing and conflicting medical opinion

▶ Organisation of medical rotas

▶ The complaints process.

Outcome

The report from the Independent Review Panel stated that they accepted that the original complaint was in 1998 and thought that it was likely that some positive changes had been made as a result of the initial investigation. However, specific recommendations were made, as follows:

1. A consultant-led post-take ward round should occur seven days a week.
2. An increase in junior staff is urgently required.
3. A medical senior registrar should be available at all times.
4. Cardiac enzyme estimations should be available on call at all times.
5. A technician-run weekend venesection service should be available.
6. A system of formal communication between one clinical firm and another should be initiated.
7. The Trust needs to agree a universal procedure for the management of acute myocardial infarction and acute ischaemia.
8. A more readily available and responsive ECG service should be provided.
9. Letters sent by the Chief Executive to a complainant but drafted by others first must be agreed with the appropriate consultants, both for factual content and accuracy. This system should be formalised.
10. Where it is obvious that there has been a clear breach of duty, the Trust should accept responsibility early, and communication with the complainant should be entirely transparent.

Action taken

This complaint led to the most major review of the management of emergency admissions, the management of complaints and the supervision of junior staff. Time will tell if the changes have the desired affect.

Case 5

Miss H, a 54-year-old lady with learning disability, was admitted to hospital for elective neurosurgery to remove a pituitary tumour. The surgery went well and her postoperative recovery was uneventful, the main concern being to ensure optimal endocrinological function. This was managed through an appropriate referral to a specialist physician. On the fifth postoperative day, the patient was visited by a relative, who took her out of the ward for a walk. Whilst she was out of the ward, Miss H fell and was brought back to the ward, having apparently sustained an injury to her upper arm. She was seen later by a junior doctor, but was not X-rayed initially. When she *was* X-rayed, she was transferred to another hospital within the same Trust, to the care of the trauma unit. The relatives were not informed of the transfer at the time.

During her time on the trauma unit, Miss H became very unwell, and was subsequently transferred again, back to the original hospital, and readmitted to a high-dependency unit under the care of the endocrinology team. Her condition was stabilised and she was eventually moved back to a medical ward for a further programme of rehabilitation. Sadly, her recovery was poor after this event, and, after a further transfer to a hospital nearer her home, she died a few months later. A relative kept a diary of events throughout Miss H's hospitalisation, the details of which make for stark reading set against the issues raised. Moreover, because the notes are missing, the allegations cannot be refuted or corroborated as the information is not available.

Issues

▶ Lack of care

▶ Lost medical notes

▶ Communication failures

▶ Care planning.

Action taken

A multidisciplinary meeting has been held with the relatives, and the questions that they raised have been dealt with honestly and openly. Although statements from clinical staff have been taken, it is very difficult to be able to refute the allegations in the light of the continuing absence of the patient's medical records. The case remains open.

Summary

All of these case studies had an element of poor communication within them; all could have been handled better and possibly could have been managed more effectively and positively – for the Trust and the complainants alike – at an earlier stage. It seems clear that there are occasions when we have to acknowledge fault and accept responsibility, without admitting liability, and work harder to ensure that we *do* learn from our mistakes through sharing case studies. The Trust in question now actively reviews cases periodically, in a multidisciplinary setting, and then the cases are used at directorate level as a learning opportunity.

In addition to the specific actions demanded as a result of the investigation of complaints, other actions have been taken to remedy complaints on the basis of an analysis of the commonly held top four classifications (diagnosis and treatment, staff attitudes, poor communication, and waiting times). The most common complaints surround diagnosis and treatment and some of the issues raised have been identified within the case studies. The following, in order, are classifications of the next highest numbers of complaints together with some action points.

Staff attitudes

Directorate training packages have been devised based on real cases that have been anonymised. The Health Service Commissioner's epitomes also are used specifically to draw out problems which occur as a result of poor staff attitudes. Individual staff members also are invited to attend meetings with complainants and to give feedback to colleagues. Customer care training is now applied across the staff groups.

Poor communication

An emphasis is placed on staff maintaining good communication – both written and verbal – through induction programmes and inhouse training. This is an ongoing problem, which, despite the best efforts, continues to be a regular problem with complainants.

Waiting times

Individual directorates are made aware of specific areas of concern through the formal performance-monitoring arrangements, contracting discussions and the requirement to furnish commissioners with key information set against agreed performance indicators.

Complaints management: What have we learnt so far?

The number of complaints continues to grow, and the Health Service Commissioner's (HSC) Office expect a 10% rise in their workload year on year. During 1998/1999, the HSC established working procedures for clinical investigations and is now open to receiving complaints about clinical judgement, and the actions of Family Health Services Authorities now will be under the jurisdiction of the HSC. There also is a steady increase in the requests for Independent Reviews, which further underlines both the public's insistence on being heard and the need to work harder on local resolution.

Complaints also appear to be becoming more complex. Complaints have a host of causes: poor training, poor communication, wrong information, high stress levels, defensiveness in managing criticism, staff perceptions, lack of priority, and inappropriate management. Consequently, if you look at the complaints that are generated over a period of time, for any organisation, the number received will vary – but they will be centred round an average, and it is the average that counts. Managers and committees who monitor complaints levels as a measure of performance must understand that variations from month to month are significant only if they deviate significantly or if there is a persistent trend. If this happens, there is a specific cause, which will need to be investigated and an action plan developed.

As described earlier, it can be demonstrated that the two most common causes of increasing numbers of complaints since 1990 have been the launch of the Patients' Charter and the implementation of the recommendations of the Wilson report,[1] both of which increased the accessibility and awareness for complainants. To have interpreted these events as a sign that there was an overall decrease in performance across the health service could have proved demoralising and led to excessively negative investigations. Such actions can foster a blame culture that discourages reports of 'near misses'. Quite simply, the NHS needs its complaints procedure to:

▶ satisfy complainants

▶ enhance the reputation of its service

▶ avoid protracted correspondence

▶ avoid unnecessary litigation

▶ use complaints as a means of improving services

▶ be fair to staff, and

▶ maintain a balance between treating staff appropriately and maintaining proper accountability for their actions.

Conclusions

Complaints can be used positively in several ways. They can provide an opportunity for providers to see themselves and their service as others see them and to identify the issues that concern users. Most importantly, complaints can allow rectification of a past mistake and enable services to be put right for the future. A well-handled complaint can increase a patients trust in doctors, nurses, other healthcare staff and managers. Finally, complaints can enable identification of adverse events that might otherwise go undetected; they also may be the 'tip of the iceberg', the indicator of a bigger or deeper problem, which can be investigated at an early stage. They can act as an early warning system for legal claims and, if properly categorised, contextualised, recorded and analysed, can identify areas for quality improvement plans.

Our aims must be to reduce the chances of a catastrophe to negligible levels and to deal effectively with the less severe but more common incidents that form the basis of most complaints. In trying to do this, there is always a temptation to concentrate on tightening policies and procedures rather that examining the organisational culture. This is because these are the tangible controls that can be audited and measured and that, in turn, restore public confidence. Clearly, these actions have their proper place, but managing risk is as much a matter of values, leadership, organisational culture and effective communications as it is about good management systems – and this must be reflected in the way complaints are handled.

Complaints often are quoted as being the source of ideas for quality improvement programmes, but there are many facets to this and there is one important question: does your organisation appreciate the potential of the complaints it receives? Understanding the implications of your complaints is central to the actions that you and your organisation take to improve quality, the messages that are given to all staff and the organisational culture that supports risk management. Complaints can provide input to support clinical audit, risk management and quality initiatives. Genuine partnerships between patients, their families and advocates and NHS staff can result.

The best of all worlds is a partnership with patients, which looks at complaints as a valued tool for improved quality – not a measure of quality improvement. Complaints should play a part in improving standards by initiating systematic review of incidents and triggering action to avoid future problems.[8] Effective handling of complaints should include learning from the situation and from preventing recurrence, in line with recent developments in clinical risk management.

A study published in July 1994[8] showed that complainants want changes to be made as a result of their experiences. The result from this study highlighted several key issues that required recognition and action if the quality 'loop' was to be closed and similar incidents avoided in future. First, the study found that most incidents stemmed from incidents that led to significant clinical consequences and distress. In many instances, deterioration in the patient's clinical condition had led to additional treatment and longer stays in hospital. Second, clinical complaints are seldom about an error of clinical judgement alone but are often about staff insensitivity and poor communication. Third, the way the complaint was handled compounded the difficulties and intensified the distress or dissatisfaction that led to the complaint in the first place. Finally, complainants often emphasise the need for more involvement in decision-making in relation to their condition and treatment and about being kept better informed about progress and problems. Simple enough, but we are back to the basics of providing adequate information, being effective communicators and accepting our roles as partners in care.

> A customer is the most important visitor on our premises. He is not dependent on us – we are dependent on him. He is not an interruption of our work, he is the purpose of it. He is not an outsider on our business – he is part of it. We are not doing him a favour by serving him – he is doing us a favour by giving us the opportunity to do so.

Mahatma Gandhi

References

1   Wilson Committee. *Being Heard*. The report of a review committee on NHS complaints procedures. London: Department of Health, 1994.
2   Kent P. Apologies are the best insurance [Letter]. *Health Service Journal* 1991, 21 March: 10.
3   Simanowitz A. Standards, attitudes and accountability in the medical profession. *Lancet* 1985; ii: 546.
4   Simanowitz A. Accountability. In: Vincent CA, Ennis M, Audley RJ, eds. *Medical Accidents*. Oxford: Oxford University Press, 1993; 209–221.
5   NHS Executive. *Complaints, Listening, Acting, Improving*. London: Department of Health, March 1996.
6   Reason JT. Understanding adverse events; human factors. *Quality in Health Care* 1995; 4: 80–89.
7   Bennett J, Walshe K. Occurrence screening as a method of audit. *BMJ* 1990; 300: 1248–1251.
8   Bark P *et al*. Clinical complaints: a means of improving the quality of care. *Quality in Health Care* 1994; 3: 123–132.

8

The Organisation and Evidence-Based Practice

Myriam Lugon

Introduction

The development and launch of a national research and development strategy[1] has raised the profile of research and highlighted the need for organisations to be more explicit about their research activities, to develop network with academic institutions and to avoid duplication of effort. This was followed by the setting up of a national research programme for which funding was identified; such as the Health Technology assessment programme,[2] which aims to ensure that costly interventions or innovations are truly evaluated before being implemented. National research priorities were identified and Regional Research and Development Directorates were given the lead for one or more of the confirmed priorities. As a result, clinical effectiveness has become part of day to day language amongst all individuals involved in healthcare as well as patient organisations; the consumer role in evidence-based healthcare has been highlighted;[3,4] and a national framework for action has been published by the NHS Executive.[5]

Clinical guidelines, supported by the NHS Executive,[6] have been identified as a key tool to promote best practice. Criteria for successful development and implementation of clinical guidelines have been published in a Nuffield Institute for Health publication in 1994.[7] Information on effective treatment and interventions has been made available through a number of sources[8] and disseminated by regional offices to Health Authorities and medical directors of Trusts (eg the North Thames resource pack). This information is often the result of systematic reviews produced in a format and language not accessible to all healthcare professionals. Dissemination of effectiveness information does not, however, guarantee changes in clinical practice. A study by Oxman[9] has shown that there is no easy recipe to implementation of research findings, which may also require funding; unfortunately, this is no longer available through the research levy.[10]

The research and effectiveness agenda has been medically dominated; Health Authorities have often required Trusts to ensure that changes in clinical practice are implemented where the evidence is deemed robust. Such examples include treatment of myocardial infarction,[11] treatment of glue ear,[12] and dilatation and curettage.[13] Again, this approach reinforces the medical domination of the agenda and ignores the fact that care is given by a clinical team and that evidence, if not always clear cut, exists for non-doctor interventions.

The importance of ensuring that patients receive treatment that is both clinically and cost-effective has been re-emphasised by establishment of the National Institute for Clinical Excellence (NICE) and the publication of National Service Frameworks (NSFs), which establish national standards and define service needs for specific care groups.[14] (NICE and clinical governance is discussed in details in chapter 11). A number of guidelines have now been published and disseminated to the NHS, and organisations are expected to ensure that clinical practice meets national standards.

Within this context, healthcare organisations have to take the research and development agenda forward as one element of improving quality of care, and ensure that the appropriate systems and processes are in place.

What is the role of the healthcare organisation?

Healthcare organisations need to foster a climate encouraging staff to ask the following questions: 'Are we doing things right?' 'What is the available evidence pertaining to my practice?' And 'How can I influence colleagues to change practice if appropriate?' Staff will need to understand what is meant by 'research and development' (R&D), and how these activities can help them in their day-to-day practice. This understanding is necessary at all levels, not only at that of the clinician but also at managerial level.[15] It must be recognised, however, that many more healthcare organisations will be involved in the development end of R&D (ie the implementation of evidence-based practice to improve patient outcomes, rather than pure biomedical research). Information on effectiveness must therefore be targeted at the appropriate specialty and its implementation monitored.

Healthcare organisations are there to ensure that the quality of care delivered is optimal to achieve excellent patient outcomes. Thus, the R&D agenda must be linked to clinical audit and risk, to the development of explicit service standards and to the education and training plan of any service. The Medical Director and board member accountable to the Chief Executive should manage these interdependent processes, and strong links should be established with the complaints department. In giving the overall management responsibility to the one individual, there will be better communication and coordination of the work undertaken and these initiatives are more likely to be taken forward harmoniously.

The Medical Director needs, on behalf of the Chief Executive, to ensure that the right systems and processes are in place to deliver effective clinical practice and improve patient care but also that managers within the Trust understand the importance of this agenda and support it even when the Health Service is under pressure. This approach is a step in the direction of fulfilling the requirements for clinical governance described in the NHS White Paper.[16] Whilst organisational leadership is necessary, the engagement of staff and their ownership of this agenda is paramount for it to be successfully implemented. Creating a multidisciplinary R&D steering group will help ensure that the organisation's R&D strategy is implemented. The group should comprise staff with a range of skills and knowledge from different professional backgrounds but must include the managers for R&D and for clinical audit and risk, as well as the Director of Medical Education. Indeed, it is important for the training and education agenda to be linked to what is deemed best practice and for training programmes to be developed accordingly. In some Trusts, a Director of R&D would have been appointed, and such an individual should chair the R&D committee.

The details of a District Trust R&D steering group is shown in Box A. The work of such a group should be extended to the identification of training needs, thus ensuring staff are equipped with the relevant skills to take evidence-based medicine forward. Membership therefore should include an education and training representative for non-medical education.

Box A. Trust R&D steering group

Aim:

To maximise contribution of R&D to achieving the Trust's objectives.

Terms of reference:

▶ To facilitate multidisciplinary and multiagency research

▶ To act as a source of advice for staffing wanting to undertake research

▶ To maximise the use of research skills, knowledge and facilities from other organisations, eg foster academic links

▶ To facilitate the implementation of the R&D strategy and monitor the work programme

▶ To link with the relevant Health Authorities for joint work to be progressed

▶ To monitor quality of research

▶ To facilitate the integration of R&D, clinical audit and risk and quality across the Trust and support the development of effectiveness training programme

Composition:

Membership includes three consultants, a Director of Medical Education, a librarian, an R&D manager, a clinical audit and risk manager, a research midwife, a nurse involved in research, a senior manager. It is chaired by the Medical Director.
Other individuals can be co-opted if appropriate and an IM&T officer asked to attend relevant meetings.

In creating an environment fostering research, organisations must ensure that the research proposals are of the highest standards and that any resource implications have been thought through at the outset to avoid projects being halted before completion. Research proposals therefore should be vetted before being submitted for ethical approval; in particular, they should be checked against a number of criteria:

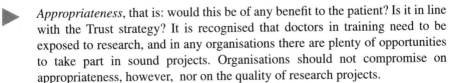 *Appropriateness*, that is: would this be of any benefit to the patient? Is it in line with the Trust strategy? It is recognised that doctors in training need to be exposed to research, and in any organisations there are plenty of opportunities to take part in sound projects. Organisations should not compromise on appropriateness, however, nor on the quality of research projects.

▶ *Quality and validity of research design,* giving particular attention to the number to be included in the project to achieve statistical significance.

▶ *Legal liability.*

▶ *Resource implications.* The cost of the research to the organisation must be identified and funding sought before the research starts – a very important step since the service cost of research needs to come out of Culyer[10] funds.

▶ *Proper accounting of income generated by research.* This is particularly important for commercially funded research to ensure that the organisation is not in breach of its statutory duties and standing financial instructions.

It is recognised that this approach may not be applicable to all organisations and may probably not be entirely appropriate for academic institutions. However, organisations with small research portfolios wanting to encourage quality research may find this approach useful. A London Trust has had in place for many years now a research approval group, which examines all research proposals. The proposals are vetted against the criteria listed above, by four to five members from different professional backgrounds, to ensure that both quantitative and qualitative research knowledge/skills are available. If queries arise, the researcher is asked for clarification and can access help and support from members of the steering group or their network. Research proposals are vetted for ethical approval before being submitted and an agreement has been reached with the local Ethics Committee, who will not consider proposals not given the go-ahead by the Trust. If such a process is set up, it is important to make the timescale for approval explicit, and to monitor the process to ensure there is no delay in approval. A framework should be developed, giving details of the process, the individual responsible for its coordination, the timetable and the relationship with the Ethics Committee. This needs to be made available to all staff undertaking research, and periodically updated and recirculated.

Research and development infrastructure

An infrastructure is necessary to manage R&D, the size of which will depend on the research agenda and portfolio, as well as on the budget of the organisation. Whilst it is accepted that academic institutions (eg teaching hospitals) will have different requirements, a district general hospital will need to ensure that they are able to foster an inquisitive culture and implement what is deemed best practice, as well as support research. A clinician to take the lead for R&D should be identified. The approach taken in one Trust described below therefore may be seen as a possible model to achieve these goals.

In this Trust, an infrastructure, both central and devolved, has been established. There is a small central R&D team comprising an R&D officer and an information officer whose responsibilities are as follows:

▶ To provide central support for research projects within the Trust (eg technical support, literature searches, brainstorming, and source of funding).

▶ To provide training in critical appraisal, thus supporting the development of a research culture.

▶ To support services in the development of guidelines and their implementation, by working closely with clinical audit staff.

▶ To disseminate effectiveness information to relevant staff, often presenting it in a more accessible format and language.

▶ To carry out specific projects using research methodologies to help in the achievement of the Trust's objectives (eg service reviews, simulation modelling, and so on).

▶ To maintain a comprehensive central database of research projects and monitor progress to assist the Trust with the Culyer requirements.

▶ To ensure the Trust is informed about the national R&D agenda and its initiatives (eg clinical effectiveness, Culyer, and calls for particular research projects).

This small team is accountable to the Clinical Governance Manager and works across organisational boundaries with the various clinical teams. A top-down approach alone, however, is unlikely to be successful if not supported by staff within given services. As such, a local R&D network is necessary; in some instances, a research unit can reinforce middle management, thus strongly linking clinical supervision to clinical effectiveness and clinical risk avoidance by ensuring that staff have the necessary skills to deliver the highest standard of care. In other services, a research nurse or midwife can take on the role of facilitating practice development and take forward relevant research projects. The overall approach is to encourage inquisitive practice by all staff, identifying standards of current practice and comparing them with national standards, providing training in search strategies and critical appraisal. This ensures that staff are equipped with the necessary skills to challenge each other's practice. It can also offer a platform for the evaluation of different models of care, engaging staff at the grass roots in the process. One of the main streams of this approach is to identify what skills are of value amongst the local R&D staff in facilitating change, and to assess the support needed to allow others to develop these skills (eg evidence-based healthcare training, decision-tree analysis training, change management, and so on). This is aimed at developing a self-perpetuating network of change agents equipped with skills to train and develop others.

Specific initiatives supporting the effectiveness agenda

A number of national initiatives have professed to progress the effectiveness agenda. Any initiatives should be evaluated so that the lessons learnt can inform other organisations' approaches, however. The evaluation of the GRiP (Getting Research in Practice) project emphasised the importance of the context – organisational and managerial – in which clinicians practice, and drew logical conclusions.[17] Opportunities to use existing systems and processes such as education and audit also were identified as a lever for change.[18] The PACE (Promoting Action on Clinical Effectiveness) project recently published its interim report,[19] which included many of the lessons the teams have learnt, such as having a realistic and balanced approach, accepting that the evidence is not always clear cut and recognising that new skills may be required.

Frontline evidence-based healthcare

Frontline evidence-based medicine projects, using a method developed at McMaster University,[20] were sponsored by the North Thames Implementation Group of the R&D Directorate. These have also been evaluated,[21] and the evaluation demonstrated that the success of this initiative is dependent upon the enthusiasm of the clinical team for the project, the availability of sound evidence and the acquisition of relevant new skills. An example from a Trust that took part in the project is given in Box B.

Box B. Frontline evidence-based project: The Maternity Unit

This project was funded by the North Thames Implementation Programme. Software and databases were acquired and included access to Medline, Cinhal and others. The Cochrane database of systematic reviews were also available. The clinical team within Maternity, including consultants, the librarian, the R&D manager and the audit team, were trained by the Kings Fund (London) and the process was based on problems faced in clinical practice. The project was successful as it had the support of the managers as well as the consultants and gave the team access to information near to where clinical activity was taking place. The benefits are described below:

▶ Staff became more confident as they were able to check queries quickly.

▶ It created an inquisitive culture in the team and fostered team working

▶ It generated enthusiasm – a midwife search clinic was established; a consultant attended the Oxford evidence-based medicine course

▶ It was used by managers as well as clinical staff to inform patients, respond to complaints and check clinical practice.

It had, however, time and resource implications.

This project offered a stand-alone system. The benefits therefore were limited to one team only. Access to effectiveness and research information should be available to all staff as and when they need it. This particular Trust pooled its resources to ensure that many more initiatives could be implemented. Such initiatives include the following:

▶ A Medline service is available to all staff; this makes explicit the principles of searching on the system and is given support by library staff.

▶ Courses in effective literature searching are run regularly; this aims to improve the awareness of the relevant databases and help staff to understand how to formulate effective search strategies by making use of the local information service. This has now been extended to include basic statistical training, basic research methodologies and decision-tree analysis. It forms part of a modular training approach available to all clinical teams and delivered whenever possible on a multidisciplinary basis. Whilst there are many critical appraisal courses, having such training on site focusing on the practical clinical problems identified by the team has many advantages. Its comprehensiveness is also of benefit; the modular basis allows a team to progress at its own pace.

► Internet project has been established. The Trust home page contains information on courses run by the Medical Education Centre and a distance-learning package for a specialist registrar in respiratory medicine has been developed.

► A computer-assisted learning centre has been established that is networked with services within the main hospital so that research information, textbook and training material are available at all times. There are 30 networked stations and one has been set up in the junior doctors' mess.

Integrated care pathways

A lot of emphasis has been put on the development of clinical guidelines as a tool to take best practice forward.[6] Healthcare professionals are, however, concerned about their legal implications,[22] and the implementation of guidelines has not been without its difficulties. Organisations thus need to ensure that clinical effectiveness is taken forward at the same time as organisational effectiveness; the development of integrated care pathways (multidisciplinary care plans) will help fulfil this need.[23] A number of integrated care pathways have been developed covering a range of clinical conditions such as fracture of the neck of the femur,[24] treatment of strokes,[25] and management of unstable angina,[26] and some Trusts have posted their pathways on the Internet. In developing pathways, organisations should build on what already exists. Successful implementation, however, needs a number of factors to be present:

► A credible member of staff able to facilitate the work

► A reasonable timescale

► The pathways documentation must replace the notes to avoid duplication

► Investment in training the clinical teams is needed

► A sound monitoring system must be in place. This highlights the importance of clinical audit as a tool to monitor effective practice.

Clinical audit

With the advent of clinical governance, monitoring clinical practice is likely to become a mandatory process for any healthcare organisations, who will need to therefore use clinical audit as a tool to demonstrate the outcome of care. It is likely that there will be a requirement to make results explicit on an annual basis. Clinical audit has not so far been wholly supported by clinicians.[27] The results of a national survey also highlighted the lack of appropriate and effective methodology.[28]

Organisations need to link firmly clinical audit to the effectiveness agenda. To avoid the pitfalls identified nationally and overcome the lack of credibility this process had within the medical profession, a robust methodology and an operational framework to systematise the key components of the audit cycle should be developed; thus firmly embedding audit within operational management. Box C describes such a framework.

Box C. A clinical audit framework

1. Identifying audit topics: the topics must be developed by the service multi-professional management team taking into account the views of staff at all levels.

2. The audit topics must take into account critical incidents, complaints and claims information as well as NICE guidance and so on.

3. Prioritising audit activities: the clinical governance committee should be involved in prioritising audit topic according to criteria such as high volume, high risk, high cost, in line with the organisation business plan and audit strategy, patient focus, clear ownership by clinical teams, etc.

4. Defining and analysing audit projects: agreements are in place between the audit service and the clinical team at the beginning of the project, clarifying roles and responsibilities.

5. Identifying and selecting solutions: audit project team presents clear conclusions to clinical teams for agreement; these are then translated into clear actions.

6. Implementing solutions: actions are taken by the appropriate lead identified at the feedback within a clear timescale. Outcome is monitored through performance management mechanism at least twice yearly.

7. Evaluating and re-auditing: snapshot audits are undertaken to monitor the implementation of audit recommendations and changes in clinical practice to ensure changes are sustained.

When developing the clinical audit programme, it is important to give the various services available and the relevant information concerning the effectiveness agenda (ie relevant effective healthcare bulletin, etc), clinical risk (ie incident and claims reports), complaints data and clinical indicators. Moreover, it is also important to state the explicit criteria, with the aim of identifying problem areas requiring further investigations. The audit programme thus can help services to improve outcomes of patient care and the quality of the service delivery.

Clinical effectiveness and the manager

All too often, managers feel they cannot interfere in matters of clinical practice. Although it would not be appropriate for any manager to dictate how patients should be treated, they do have a role to play in taking this agenda forward.[29] Firstly, they need to support the development of an inquisitive and learning culture to improve quality of care. They also need to ensure that staff have the appropriate skills to deliver that care and then ensure that these needs are included in the service training plan and accept clinical effectiveness as an integral part of routine practice. It must be recognised, however, that evidence is not always clear cut and should not be used as a tool to cut costs. Managers should also accept that clinical practice issues can be used to develop clinical indicators that can become part of the performance review and an integral part of operational management. As clinicians are increasingly taking on management roles, this is becoming more and more important; and it is necessary as Chief Executives take on statutory responsibility for quality of care.[15] Managers also should recognise that the effectiveness agenda cannot stand alone but must be part of a process of continuous clinical improvement linking clinical audit, risk, standards, complaints and education. Chief Executives, supported by their medical and nursing directors, will need to consider whether their organisational framework fosters this integration. A board-level director must be given the responsibility to take this agenda forward, but support from management colleagues must be forthcoming.

Effecting change in clinical practice is not a quick and easy process; it requires time, support and facilitation – at times even resources. The organisation must be prepared to support clinicians in their endeavour to improve patient outcomes and ensure that implementation of research findings occur.

Challenges faced by organisations

Talking about clinical effectiveness and evidence-based practice can be a turn off for many professionals. Clinicians are trained to do their best for their patients and have a duty to keep up to date.[30] The information available is not always couched in a language accessible to all. A common language must therefore be used and jargon avoided. This may require the translation of published material into simple bullet-point statements before being disseminated widely. It also is important to ensure that initiatives supporting the effectiveness agenda are truly multidisciplinary, allowing for clinical teams to develop together and thus ensuring that professional barriers are broken down.

Work within this field will enhance the reputation of a department or specialty and thus facilitate the recruitment and retention of staff as well as influencing users – lay and professional – of services. Sound clinical audit, robust clinical risk management systems and the ability to learn from complaints, incidents etc., if in place and effective, are likely to place services ahead in the achievement of the clinical governance requirements. Finally, the production of national guidelines – compliance with which is required to obtain accreditation to treat certain types of patients – can provide an important driver of changes, as seen with the Calman–Hine initiatives in cancer services,[31] and, more recently, in the treatment of cancer of the colon[32] and lung.[33] This approach is likely to continue, as highlighted in the NHS White Paper.[34]

Quality monitoring

The White Paper[34] has placed quality as a new responsibility of Chief Executives. Appropriate mechanisms therefore must be in place to ensure that care given is both clinically and cost-effective, and that clinical governance requirements are met.[35] Clinical effectiveness is only one aspect of improvement in clinical practice; the organisational framework thus must cover all aspects (eg risk, complaints, effectiveness and NICE guidance, audit, education and training), and must demonstrate that the clinical teams are able to effect changes having reflected on their day-to-day practice.[36] This requires a new approach to performance review of clinical services.

Conclusion

To move the clinical effectiveness agenda forward successfully in any organisation, a real partnership between all key players must be struck – from the grass roots to the Chief Executive. Managers must be part of the process. Good working relationships will need to be developed, as well as effective internal and external networks. A climate fostering an inquisitive learning culture must be created and enthusiasm generated. This needs an organisational approach, led by the Chief Executive, the identification of champions and the development of a critical mass of staff to support the process. Only then can an organisation truly become a learning one, and begin to fulfil the requirements of clinical governance.

References

1   Research for Health. Department of Health. London, September 1991.
2   NHS Executive. The Annual Report of the NHS Health Technology Assessment Programme 1997. Identifying Questions, Finding Answers. Leeds: Department of Health, 1997.
3   Hyatt J. In It Together: Promoting Information for Shared Decision Making. London: Kings Fund, 1997.
4   Promoting Action on Clinical Effectiveness (PACE), Involving Patients. PACE Bulletin. September (special issue) 1996; 1–4.
5   NHS Executive. Promoting Clinical Effectiveness: a Framework For Action in and Through the NHS. Leeds, 1996.
6   NHS Management Executive. Improving Clinical Guidelines, EL(93)115. Leeds: Department of Health, 1993.
7   Nuffield Institute for Health. Effective Health Care. Implementing Clinical Guidelines, Bulletin No. 8. Leeds: University of Leeds, 1994.
8   Miles A, Lugon M (eds). Effective Clinical Practice. Appendix: Available Information on Clinical Effectiveness, 248–249. Oxford: Blackwell Science, 1996.
9   Oxman AD, Thomson MA, Davis DA, Haynes RB. No magic bullet: a systematic review of 102 trials of intervention to improve clinical practice. Canadian Medical Association Journal 1995; 153: 1423–1431.
10 Culyer DA. Supporting Research and Development in the NHS. London: HMSO, 1994.

11 Fibrinolytic Therapy Trialists Group. Indications for fibrinolytic therapy in suspected acute myocardial infarction: collaborative overview of early mortality and major morbidity results from all randomised trials of more than 1000 patients. *Lancet* 1994; 343: 11–22.

12 Nuffield Institute for Health. *Effective Healthcare. Treatment of Persistent Glue Ear in Children*, Bulletin No. 4 Leeds: University of Leeds, 1992.

13 Nuffield Institute for Health. *The Management of Menorrhagia*, Bulletin No. 9. Leeds: University of Leeds, 1995.

14 *A First Class Service. Quality in the NHS*. London: Department of Health, HSC 1998/113.

15 Dunning M, Lugon M, MacDonald J. Clinical effectiveness. Is clinical effectiveness a management issue? *BMJ* 1998; 316: 243–244.

16 DoH. *The New NHS – Modern. Dependable*. London: The Stationary Office, 1997. Lugon M, Secker-Walker J (eds). Integrated care. In *Clinical Governance. Making It Happen*. London: RSM Press, 1999: 47.

17 Dopsons S, Gabbey J. *Getting Research into Practice and Purchasing Issues and Lessons from Four Countries*. Anglia and Oxford RHA, 1996.

18 Murphy M, Dunning M. Implementing clinical effectiveness – is it time for a change of gear? *British Journal of Health Care Management* 1997; 3(1): 243–244.

19 Dunning M, Abi-Aad G, Gukbert D, Gillam S, Livett H. *Turning Evidence into Everyday Practice*. London: Kings Fund, 1998.

20 Rosenberg W, Donald A. Evidence based medicine. An approach to clinical problem solving. *BMJ* 1995; 310: 1122–1126.

21 Donnald A. *The Front Line Evidence Based Medicine Project – Final Report*. London: NHS Executive North Thames Regional Office, Research & Development, 30 June 1998.

22 Hurwitz B. The authority and legal standing of clinical standards and practice guidelines. In: Miles A, Lugon M (eds.) *Effective Clinical Practice*. 205–225. Oxford: Blackwell Science, 1996.

23 Campbell H. Integrated care pathways. *BMJ* 1998; 316: 133–137.

24 Ogilvie-Harris DJ, Hawk RW. Elderly patients with hip fractures improved outcome with the use of care maps with high quality medical and nursing protocols. *Journal of Orthopaedic Trauma* 1993; 7: 428–437.

25 Sulch D, Kalra L. *The Role of Integrated Care Pathways in the Implementation of Effective Practice into Mainstream Care*. Stroke Rehabilitation Unit based in a district general hospital, 2000. See URL: www.doh.gov.uk/ntrd/rd/reimplem/complete/kalr.htm.

26 Catherwood E, O'Rourke DJ. Critical pathway management of unstable angina. *Progress in Cardiovascular Disease* 1994; 3: 121–148

27 McKee M. Is money wasted on audit? *Journal of the Royal Society of Medicine* 1994; 87: 52–55.

28 Buttery J, Walsh K, Coles Y, Bennet J. *Evaluating Medical Audit: The Development of Audit – Findings of a National Survey of Healthcare Provider Units in England*. London: Caspe Research, 1994.

29 Burke C, Lugon M. Integrating clinical risk and clinical audit – moving towards clinical governance. *Healthcare Risk Resource* 1998; 2:16–18.

30 General Medical Council. Duties of a Doctor and Good Medical Practice. London: 1998.

31 DoH and Welsh Office. *A Policy Framework for Commissioning Cancer Services*, 1995.

32 NHS Executive. *Guidance on Commissioning Cancer Services. Improving the Outcomes in Colorectal Cancer*. Leeds: Department of Health, 1997.

33 NHS Executive. *Guidance on Commissioning Cancer Services. Improving the Outcomes in Lung Cancer*. Leeds: Department of Health, 1998.

34 Department of Health. *The New NHS. Modern. Dependable. The National Dimension*. Leeds, 1997: 55–62.

35 Lugon M. Secker-Walker J. Organisational framework for clinical governance. In: *Clinical Governance. Making it Happen*. London: RSM Press, 1999: 15–31.

36 Department of Health. *The New NHS. Modern. Dependable. Driving Performance*. Leeds, 1997: 48–49.

▶9

The Myth of Accurate Clinical Information

Nicola Roderick, Alan Roderick

Introduction

In order to deliver the clinical governance agenda, good quality, timely, accurate information is needed to establish baselines and to enable ongoing monitoring against standards and benchmarks.

Such information is not always available or accurate, and is rarely owned by clinicians. There are many problems surrounding information that need to be resolved in order to fully support the clinical governance process and shift the focus of information from a management and financial tool towards an electronic patient record (EPR). Information collection and analysis needs to be adequately resourced and planned. Robust systems need to be implemented, with key stakeholders being involved at every stage. There are many challenges for the future and much investment needed; changes are required in the very culture of the NHS.

Clinical governance, whilst a long-term agenda, is happening now, however. National clinical indicators are being published based on existing data. This same data also will be used to report on the National Performance Frameworks. The Commission for Health Improvement (CHI) also access Trust data prior to their visits, and thus Trusts need to try to make good use of the information currently available to them. They need to share it within the organisation, encourage ownership and discussion, take data quality issues seriously, and start to change the culture. Certainly, at national level – both in England and Wales – there is recognition of the need to satisfy the information requirements of healthcare professionals. The information management and technology (IM&T)/information strategies for both England and Wales make it clear that the information needs of healthcare professionals, as well as the public, patients, managers and planners, are expected to be met during the 1998–2005 time period.

Information required must be specified correctly, produced accurately and interpreted correctly. Unfortunately, the track record of the NHS is poor in these aspects. There are fundamental weaknesses, both in terms of understanding and dealing with information and also in terms of interpreting requirements and translating those requirements into meaningful results.

Analytical skills are not valued highly within the NHS and so there is little wonder that they are not especially prevalent. There remain inaccuracies, which undermine the process of trying to convince the NHS that investment is required. If value cannot be added through the use of information, for whatever reason, investment is unlikely. The challenge must be to derive value from existing information sources whilst clearly identifying the inherent weaknesses.

NHS management, both clinical and non-clinical, demands that information produced is robust and available in an instant. Whilst this in itself is not unreasonable, the fact that there is limited acknowledgement from these two groups that they have an essential and non-negotiable role to play in this process gives an insight into why the process is failing.

Information for Health. An Information Strategy for the Modern NHS 1998–2005[1] makes it perfectly clear that there is a lack of understanding amongst NHS managers that information and information technology is a critical chief executive issue and is not the preserve of the IT specialist. Strategists should know, however, that this has been the case for many years and that it will not be possible to change this situation without a clear lead, from the highest level.

Clinical information

> A clinical information system can be defined as one which will contain all the administrative, demographic and person-based information relating to an individuals health care which the clinician needs, when and where needed, to provide relevant, evidence-based care to that patient. The aggregate information that is derived from this enables the clinician to manage and review the quality of the clinical service provided ... Management information can then be extracted and derived from these systems without introducing burdensome data collection procedures on clinical staff, as has happened in the past. Implementing systems, which truly support clinical activity, should be the main focus for IM&T activities in provider organisations.

This definition of a clinical information system and related data is from the *Better Information – Better Health. Information Management and Technology for Health Care and Health Improvement in Wales,*[2] a strategic document produced by the Welsh Office. This definition, while similar to that in Information for Health, better emphasises the importance of clinical staff in this process. However, the strategies are not specific about what clinical information should be collected.

What information is required to support clinical governance? This undoubtedly will have to evolve over the coming years. It will vary between different, and even within, specialties. It will have to accommodate clinical indicators and the National Performance Framework. It will have to enable better audit, and be comparable with other institutions. It will have to inform and reassure Trust boards. Above all, it must be based on the information that clinicians need.

Clinical governance may be happening now, but over 75% of Trusts have not yet invested in 'clinical information systems'. So where is the information being used for the clinical indicators currently coming from? What other information is available within Trusts that could be used to aid in the clinical governance process and what needs to be done to ensure its quality?

History

The main information systems of most Trusts have evolved primarily to service the need for contract monitoring. The introduction of the GP fundholding scheme in England and Wales in the early 1990s made it necessary to collect information about patient activity to ensure that minimum data sets could be provided to GP fundholders and Health Authorities to justify the activity levels and the accompanying charges.

At that time, hospitals did not always have information departments, and if they did they were in their infancy with few technical skills. They were tasked with meeting statutory requirements such as providing minimum data sets to GP fundholders and statistical information to Health Authorities and government. The minimum data sets contained patient demographic details and basic information about the patient's stay, such as admission and discharge details, mode of admission/ discharge, and diagnosis and procedure codes. Whilst some of the information produced from the data may have been incidentally of interest to the clinical staff, it was a relatively small proportion of what was produced because the systems were not designed to collect clinical information.

Unfortunately, the purpose for which information was collected did colour the data that were collected. Contracting raised awareness of data that were not being collected – particularly if it represented activity that could be charged to a Health Authority or GP fundholder. In some cases, it persuaded Trusts to reclassify some activity in order to ensure that they were remunerated. It also raised the awareness of coding in a very limited way. Both Trusts and GP fundholder practices became very aware of the procedure codes that led to an invoice. It was not unknown for managers, accountants or clinicians to try to persuade the coding departments to use certain codes to increase revenue. Conversely, GPs would often try to argue for a primary procedure code for a patient that was not chargeable.

Information departments evolved in the various hospitals because of the need to meet the various statutory and contracting information requirements. The only data available usually came from a patient administration system. Although this could be used to produce a limited amount of 'clinical' information, this was generally secondary in importance to the statutory requirements, and the departments were not staffed to meet any clinical information needs.

To address the clinical information shortfall, the more technologically minded of the clinical staff started to procure or build their own systems. This usually occurred in a piecemeal fashion, tailored to the needs of the specific areas and without reference or linkage to the main hospital administration systems and associated staff groups. Such systems were not used for statutory reporting and were used mainly within the confines of the particular department.

Now that the NHS internal market has been modified, in theory the level of bureaucracy and paper-chasing should reduce and this should divert resources away from the production of simple, though time-consuming, contracting information. Three-year agreements between organisations in theory should release resources to concentrate on providing information in support of the clinical processes, and management information would become a 'byproduct'. This is what is being proposed strategically at a national level and is precisely what the NHS should be doing.

Although it is early days, there is already evidence to suggest that these 'long-term agreements' are in fact contracts with a slightly different 'hat'. Furthermore, as the contracting culture is very much with us, there is a risk that this culture will pervade the local health groups, primary care groups and Specialist Health Commissions, creating just as much, if not more, bureaucracy as in the past. This will result in IM&T resources concentrating once again on non-clinical information, which will be to the detriment of clinical governance.

System developments

Whilst the ideal in the NHS would be to have one large hospital system that supplied all needs, the environment is far too complex for such a system to be developed easily. The need for any system usually runs ahead of strategy and many years ahead of funding. As a result, most Trusts have many different information systems that have been developed in a piecemeal fashion as needs have arisen. Most patient administration systems are commercial products, and have limited functionality. Major systems for areas such as theatres, radiology, pathology and pharmacy are normally purchased separately. Within one Trust, all the previously mentioned systems could be obtained from different suppliers. The compatibility problems that arise from this situation are compounded by Trust mergers and reconfigurations, which increase the numbers of different systems in use within one organisation.

There also may be many smaller systems to support the needs of individual specialities. The growth of 'stand alone' clinical systems is understandable given the previous lack of an integrated clinical system development programme. However, such systems do not always contain standard patient identifiers, and are usually used in isolation from each other and the main hospital administration systems. This leads to the duplication of information input. There is limited access to these systems outside the local area. They may use standard coding classifications but do not have trained coders inputting such information, or they may have developed their own coding systems without any reference to standard classifications and usage. Many are developed without reference to the IT department, by staff members or contractors. There are usually no service agreements and no support for such systems in future years. They do not always use the standard data definitions, and this makes it even more difficult to try to unite data from various systems to aid in clinical audit.

These create many administrative problems. Most Trusts do not have the appropriate processes in place to keep all these different systems synchronised. If somewhere in the process of treatment a change of address or name is received, it is rarely reflected in all relevant systems. It is quite probable that it will not even be known in which systems the patients are recorded.

Some of these systems are guarded jealously by the areas that own them, and data shared with other users grudgingly. There are often good reasons, however, for this defensive position. Staff acquainted with the data know the pitfalls of interpretation and also that data supplied for one purpose is often used for another. Whilst this is understandable, it is detrimental in the longer term. As these systems all exist in isolation, the understanding of the differences between them and why the same query answered from different systems may produce different results are seldom questioned. The relative data quality of these systems is never explored. These sorts of comparisons are made only under great time pressure for specific issues, and very rarely followed up again at a later date. Whenever adverse results are published from hospital administration systems, these local departmental systems are used as a means of disputing the figures. This process is reactive, not proactive, and is ultimately destructive.

Ideally, each Trust should create a clinical information committee for cross-education about these various systems. This should be used to test and improve data quality in the various systems, and to ensure that a consistent patient master index is being maintained. Such a committee also could be used to look for ways to provide hybrid information using data from more than one of the systems. This would open up new analysis possibilities, for instance, linking the basic outcome information from the main administration system to theatre data. This would enable Trusts to reap some of the analysis benefits of the EPR now. In the longer term, such a committee could help to inform the development of the EPR.

Clinical coding and quality

The standard classifications

Clinical coding is, perhaps, a misleading term. The mandatory coding systems of OPCS-4 (Classification of Surgical Operations and Procedures) and ICD-10 (International Statistical Classification of Diseases and Related Health Problems) in current usage in minimum data sets are statistical rather than clinical. However, followed properly, such classifications do allow the comparison of data collected in various hospitals, and do provide some information about the care of a patient in a hospital. Although they may not suit every area, they are not without use; they can be used to analyse clinical care, even though this analysis may be limited.

OPCS-4 is a four-digit alphanumeric classification. Each code has an alpha prefix, which identifies either the whole or part of a body system. For example 'C' is eye, 'G', the upper digestive tract, and 'W' other bones and joints. The first three digits give a general description of the type of procedure – for example, W06 represents total excision of bone. The final digit identifies the procedure more specifically – for example, W06.5 represents total excision of bone of foot nec. Most three-digit classifications include 'other specified' and 'unspecified' subcategorisations.[3]

ICD-10 is also a four-digit alphanumeric classification. Each alpha prefix describes either a particular body system disease/disorder – eg 'J' represents diseases of respiratory system – or a type of disease/disorder – eg 'C' represents neoplasms, and 'F', mental and behavioural disorders. The first three digits give a general description of the type of disease/disorder – for example, J44 represents chronic obstructive pulmonary disease; and the final digit further identifies the disease – eg J440 represents chronic obstructive pulmonary disease with acute lower respiratory infection. Again, there are usually 'other specified' and 'unspecified' subcategories also.[4]

Most clinicians do not like to use the classifications discussed above and find them restrictive and unfamiliar. The development of clinical terms (read codes) allows the capture of diagnostic and procedural information from a clinical perspective, which can then be translated back into ICD-10 and OPCS-4. Clinical terms (version 3) is due to be introduced as the standard for operational clinical systems in the UK and is supported by *Information for Health.*[1] Clinical terms not only hold codes for diseases and operations, but also encompass clinical findings and presenting symptoms.

There are plans to ensure international comparability in the future. SNOMED (systematised nomenclature of medicine) clinical terms is a joint development by the NHS and the College of American Pathologists (CAP), and will combine SNOMED RT (CAP's systematised nomenclature of medicine – reference terminology) and Clinical terms version 3. This is intended to become an essential component of EPR, and will be developed over the next five years.

ICD-10 and OPCS-4 are rapidly approaching ten years of age. Since they were published, practice has moved on, with new conditions being diagnosed and new procedures (for instance, laser surgery) being carried out. Amendments for ICD-10 are due to be implemented by April 2001, although there are very few new codes. However, coders are restricted to the classifications, and therefore have to make the best match for a particular diagnoses/condition. As Clinical terms maps back to these classifications, accuracy in analysis will continue to be impacted.

Coding quality

The use of the OPCS-4 and ICD-10 coding classifications is mandatory in the minimum data sets of Trusts' patient administration systems. However, the process of correctly collecting and recording such information is fraught with difficulty.

The process can go wrong from the very start. The staff responsible for recording events and diagnoses in the patient notes are usually busy junior doctors, and not their more experienced consultant colleagues. Those writing in the patient notes do not always understand the significance of such information for other purposes, not just for the patient, but for measuring performance. Events/diagnoses can go unrecorded, or if present are often recorded illegibly. Sometimes, conflicting diagnoses are recorded without any further explanation. Bad filing can make it extremely difficult for coders to find enough information – they sometimes have to code from scraps of paper, not notes. Whilst coders have rigorous rules to follow about how they should code from the notes, clinical statements are not presented in a way that makes these rules easy to follow. Notes may not be available because they have been sent to the coroner, or they may not have been signed out of the library and are therefore temporarily (or even permanently) lost.

In the past especially, coders did not always have access to clinicians to check or query comments in the notes. There is usually little time to code each set of notes and the clinical staff have pressing time schedules which mean that they cannot revisit the coding. Coding is often rushed to meet local and/or regional deadlines. All these pressures will affect the quality of the coding produced. In addition, coders are often based in obscure parts of the hospital, giving them little profile. Many clinical staff are unaware of what the coders do or who they are, unless of course they are either extremely enthusiastic about data or they have tried to exert undue influence on the coders in the past to change the way in which they code.

Until recently, the importance of having trained coders was not always understood.

To ensure comparability between coded information everywhere, all coders need to be fully trained in the usage of ICD-10 and OPCS-4 and to keep up to date with central guidance and coding rules. They must always comply with the coding rules, and local deviations from recommended practice must be avoided. The use of unspecified codes should be monitored carefully. Coders must ensure that they code all relevant co-morbidities to ensure that the complexity of patients is reflected accurately. However, it is important also to ensure that they do not 'overcode' a record by including conditions relating to an earlier episode that have no bearing on the management of the patient in the current episode. They should avoid coding signs and symptoms rather than diagnoses. The systems used for the inputting of coding must have adequate validation. They should not allow coding 'errors', such as the placing of laterality codes in the primary position, or the incorrect use of dagger and asterix (aetiology and manifestation) codes.

Coders need to be recognised and respected as a profession, to work with other coders, and be supervised by trained coders. At present, however, coders are still usually relatively poorly paid in spite of the growing recognition of the importance of coding. This affects the calibre and/or commitment of staff attracted into coding jobs, as well as determining how long they are likely to stay in such posts. Part of the necessary information culture change in the NHS does involve building relationships between clinicians and coders, and providing opportunities for discussions about complex cases. The feeding back of coded information to the clinicians should also raise awareness of coding problems.

There is a need for consistency in coding between coders within a Trust and between Trusts to ensure comparability of data. Quality indicators must be monitored within each Trust, and used as indicators of relative coding quality between Trusts. Typical indicators of coding quality are as follows:

▶ Average number of codes per episode

▶ Frequency of 'ungroupable' DRG (diagnosis-related group) or HRG (healthcare resource group) codes

▶ Incidence of unspecified/non-specified codes (ie not coding to the required level of specificity)

▶ Use of signs and symptoms codes as primary diagnoses.

An independent analysis of coding quality following the Scottish practice would be the ultimate guarantor of coding quality and comparability, however. Under this system, 1% of all notes for patient activity occurring within a given year are checked independently against the coding, and thus inter-Trust comparisons can be made.

There also has been debate as to whether or not clinical staff themselves should be coding. Whilst it is arguable that they would know exactly what happened to the patients, they also would have to submit to coding discipline to ensure consistency within and between Trusts. There is no room for 'doing your own thing', and evidence to date suggests that conformity would not rest easy with clinicians. Without consistency, however, all benchmarking information is of little use.

Casemix and benchmarking

'Casemix is the allocation of patients by type, diagnosis and treatment into iso-resource groups such as Health Care Resource Groups.'[5] HRGs have been used in England since 1994 and DRGs in Wales since 1995. From April 2000 onwards, Wales also will move to HRGs. While these groups have mainly been used for costing activities in the past, they are supposed to be meaningful clinically and are being increasingly accepted by the clinical profession.

Such grouping of activity allows more meaningful comparisons of activity to be made. Usually, the data that are recorded about the tens of thousands of patients who pass through a Trust each year makes each patient unique. However, it is not possible to analyse aggregate patient activity at so detailed a level. Casemix groups place similar patients together and therefore makes analysis easier. It also allows for more accurate benchmarking to be carried out between Trusts. It provides a mechanism for identifying Trusts who deal with more complex patients, and enables adjustment for these factors.

These groups are based on routinely collected data, including the ICD-10 and OPCS-4 codes, plus some other basic patient stay information such as age, length of stay and discharge method. However, good quality ICD-10 and OPCS-4 coding is essential for the groups to be truly useful. If incomplete information is available in the notes or the coders do not record enough relevant conditions in enough detail, this could result in the failure to identify complications in the derived HRG/DRG. Conversely, overcoding – ie the inclusion of irrelevant diagnoses – can give a misleading impression of the complexity of a patient.

The ultimate irony that can result from a failure to understand the relative quality of coding between organisations is that a Trust with good coding quality can appear to perform badly in comparative data simply because it codes adverse events when others fail to do so. All benchmarking data therefore should have a reliable data quality index to ensure that incorrect conclusions cannot be drawn.

Quality control

Controlling the quality of information is an uphill task. Whilst everyone pays lip-service to the importance of good quality information, there is a great reluctance to resource information collection functions adequately and to act upon identified problems and errors. Usually, it appears that everyone thinks it is someone else's problem. Education, communication and ownership at all levels of the organisation are essential to facilitate cultural change.

The data collection process

Whilst there always has been a broad agreement on the importance of collecting accurate data, there also seems to be a universal perception that it is somebody else's problem. In reality, such problems can be caused by the following reasons:

- Grade of staff inputting data
- Staff have other priorities
- Failure to train staff adequately
- Inadequate system front-end validation
- Failure to make information available for inputting
- Failure of Trust management to take such issues seriously.

Usually, there is a failure to understand how difficult it is to collect even the relatively simple data contained in the standard minimum data sets accurately. Hospitals are very complex environments, and patients can have many different entry and exit points to the system. How do you ensure that *every* patient who comes through the door has their demographic and GP details checked and any amendments entered onto the central system? How do you track all ward and consultant changes? Given the complexity of healthcare, it is surprising perhaps that the data is as accurate as it is.

However, the quality of data is only as good as the staff responsible for input. Often, staff do not have sufficient education in the importance and uses of the data, leading to the tendency to use 'bucket' codes or even misuse fields. Such misuse can go on for years and be discovered quite by accident. The effect on information, however, can be profound.

It is possible that the demands on the staff compete with the needs of patients and therefore never appear to be important. Sometimes, the information necessary for input to the system is not available at the time of input. There is also a continual expectation at management level that additional data can be recorded without any increase in staff numbers.

Whatever systems are used for collecting data, they must have appropriate front-end validation controls to ensure that conflicting or nonsense data cannot be entered. Input screens should be clear and easy to read. They also should produce regular exception reports on data that are subjective or anomalous, for review. There should be an audit trail identifying an individual user for every data item, so that identified problems can be traced back to source and remedied.

Outcomes data

Currently, collected data are of limited use when trying to measure the quality of care patients receive whilst in hospital. The standard minimum data set only identifies whether or not a patient has died in hospital, and where they have been discharged to (ie at home, in a nursing home or other NHS acute hospital). A day-surgery patient dying at home of a pulmonary embolism three days post-operatively would not be recorded on the hospital information system, for example.

Clinicians would like to know whether or not patients die after leaving hospital if the death is related to the condition the patient was treated for. They should know if the patients' quality of life has improved, and whether or not the treatment administered was effective. They need to be able to audit the outcomes of various forms of treatments to decide whether or not they are effective and worthwhile. This information is not available in hospital systems, and it will only be the advent of an integrated EPR and electronic healthcare record that will enable the sharing of such information across both primary and secondary care.

Ensuring quality

Whilst it is important to have formal mechanisms in place for monitoring data quality, many problems are uncovered inadvertently. Information departments and others carrying out data analysis often highlight anomalies, and good systems managers will often identify errors in their daily work. Unfortunately, there are not always the resources to follow through and investigate thoroughly.

One of the most useful quality checks on data is through feeding it back to the people who have generated the data in the first instance. Clinicians should have a fair idea of the numbers of patients they admit with particular conditions. There may be disagreement initially, but this process of reconciling the data with their perceptions is essential to promote clinical ownership of the data.

Information for Health[1] states that the data accreditation process will be mandatory from 2000/2001 in the acute sector. This information will be reported routinely to Trust boards. These national initiatives to improve data quality are extremely welcome; however, it is vital that too much is not expected too soon. To date, only seven Trusts in England have achieved data accreditation and although there is an ambitious plan in Wales for all Trusts to be accredited by 31 March 2001, this is unlikely to happen. Even so, if a data quality programme were to be implemented in 2001/2002, for example, this should have a positive effect on a proportion of 2001/2002 data and hence information for that year. For any meaningful clinical indicator type analysis, at least three years' data will be required. This means that it will be 2004 before robust, comparative clinical information is available throughout the NHS based on accredited data, assuming all organisations are working to the same timetable.

Ownership of data

The fact that most information existed to support contracting and not to satisfy clinical needs alienated the clinical fraternity from the start. Whilst money was not readily made available to fund clinical information systems, information about patients was being collated to assess whether or not financial requirements were being met.

Clinicians rarely were consulted, informed or involved in the data collection process, and had no idea of how or where their treatment of a patient turned into a coded record. They naturally were suspicious of a process that was invisible to them and there were seldom regular feedback mechanisms to make them acquainted with what is being stored on their patients.

As a result, clinicians have never 'owned' the data collected on the hospital administration system. Therefore, the first reaction, especially when presented with a report that appears to show something adverse, is to rubbish the data. As the information is not in frequent use within the clinical areas, it is possible that data may not be accurate. However, perceptions can often differ from reality. It also is possible that this may not be a data quality problem but rather a lack of understanding about what the information shows and how it is interpreted.

This lack of ownership will not improve if information is not widely disseminated. This will bring its own set of challenges. Some of these – for example, the dissatisfaction with the coding classifications – will not be easy to address in the short term. However, perceptions about activity levels, length of stay and numbers of patients who died can be verified to independent sources such as ward registers and patient notes. Again, the problem will be the lack of resources for this sort of detailed verification.

From data to information

'Forty two!' yelled Loonquawl. 'Is that all you've got to show for seven and a half million years' work?'

'I checked it very thoroughly,' said the computer, 'and that quite definitely is the answer. I think the problem, to be quite honest with you, is that you've never actually known what the question is.'

'But it was the Great Question! The Ultimate Question of Life, the Universe and Everything,' howled Loonquawl.

'Yes,' said Deep Thought with the air of one who suffers fools gladly, 'but what actually is it?'

The Hitch Hikers Guide to the Galaxy[6]

It is not enough to have good data collection processes in place. Data are the raw material from which information is created, and there is much information produced that does not answer any questions or help the organisation to progress. Many of the failures to turn data into information stem from communication problems within the organisation.

Data are stored with very precise definitions of the various data items; however, these are not always understood to mean the same things by management, clinicians, information analysts and the data-input staff. There are responsibilities for all parties here:

▶ The data-input staff must be educated about what the data is used for.

▶ The information department and the data-input staff must have a common understanding of how data is recorded.

▶ The information department must be explicit when passing on information to clinicians and managers about the criteria used for extracting the data and any factors that influence the result.

▶ Clinicians and management must define their queries clearly and keep both the information department and the data-input staff informed about changes in working practice and new developments.

It is extremely important to ask the right questions in order to get the information required. Sometimes, it appears that clinicians and managers expect to be given the right information when they do not actually know the question; at other times, they just do not communicate effectively. There is often a 'Chinese whisper' approach to information requests. A senior manager or clinician asks their assistant to ask their secretary to ring the information department and ask for some information without also passing along the understanding about why the information is needed or what it is expected to prove. The message has many opportunities to get diluted and misconstrued. The data that are produced does not answer the question or prove the point, or does not fit the purpose. Either the producers of the information are blamed, or the data are (once again) ridiculed.

There not only is a need to ask the right questions, however. One of the major problems with interpreting information is putting it into context. It is important to know that half the beds on a ward were closed for a period of time when completing any sort of activity analysis or calculating occupancy levels. However, there rarely are formal mechanisms in place within the organisation to ensure that the appropriate people are made aware of such events.

The development of a common language and common understanding will be of the utmost importance when defining the EPR. As the ideal is to capture data at point of contact, this means that all clinicians, nursing staff and PAMs (professionals allied to medicine) must have an equivalent understanding of how their data is recorded, and exactly what it means.

The role of the information department

The role of an information professional in the NHS is not a comfortable one. Medical records departments can feel intimidated by the continuous data checking. The IT department can sometimes resent skilled and demanding network and software users. Managers are quick to blame the department for errors in the data over which it has no control. Clinicians are suspicious of the data because they do not own it, and can object to such information being made available to managers. The department is seldom told about changes in the organisation to help interpretation of the data, or so that corrections to processes can be made. Information may be used as a political weapon by many different factions. Whilst everyone pays lip-service to information being the backbone of any organisation, it is, in reality, a largely maligned and misunderstood profession.

Whilst no one would want the doctor's receptionist to diagnose their condition, there is a popular misconception that information analysis either can be performed by low-paid administrative staff or by anyone who happens to be available. People without knowledge of how information is stored, or any knowledge of the processes in the hospital, are asked to compile figures that are used for business cases, service analyses, etc. This is not a criticism of individuals, but rather of the organisational lack of understanding about the need for individuals with the correct analytical skills to be nurtured, involved and kept informed.

As previously discussed, information departments evolved initially to meet the need for contracting and other statutory information. They have never been resourced or required to meet the clinical information need. The statutory demands on their time have not diminished, and yet clinical governance brings a whole new set of demands and reporting requirements. If a quality service is expected for the clinicians, consideration has to be given to allocating adequate resources to the job. Information staff then may be able to suggest/offer other forms of analysis to help with the process. However, the nature of the analysis of clinical information is different from contracting. A whole new set of analysis skills needs to be acquired whilst working more closely with clinicians. Information has not been perceived as a profession, where education and experience are important.

Information for Health[1] notes that 'the NHS will need to increase its current investment in specialist IM&T and clinical informatics personnel both to deliver and then exploit the investments in new technology'. This is a clear indication that there is national recognition of the need for an evolutionary approach to the delivery of information services. There is also recognition of the importance of informatics skills in clinical education. *The Education, Training and Development Strategy*,[7] which supports *Information for Health*[1] provides 'policy-level guidance about what needs to be done to help develop new skills and change the culture of information management and use in the NHS'. Analysis of health conditions and events is complex and requires continued investment in analytical skills at a local level, supported by a national infrastructure.

The future

It is not clear how the NHS will move from its current situation to achieving the goals set out in the respective strategic documents. As is nearly always the case, the stark reality of the *status quo* is rarely emphasised in high-level strategic documents. Although this is understandable, it can have several effects:

▶ Existing weaknesses will be 'glossed over', which will have to be addressed if progress is to be made.

▶ Scepticism of the ability of the NHS to deliver the strategic aims will be encouraged.

▶ Promises are made to groups of users which, in reality, may well be impossible to deliver, thus losing the audience.

▶ The strategy may be turned into a 'book-end' or 'door-stop'.

An example of an existing weakness is that the current clinical indicator publications are based on minimum data sets that have been collected nationally for over nine years. However, the initial reports produced in support of this process have resulted in waves of criticism, as a result of both quality and definitional issues.

It must be pointed out the qualitative clinical reporting from such data sets is a relatively new initiative, although long overdue. There is considerable value in collating data nationally for all organisations and ensuring that such data are comparable and of sufficient quality. Admittedly, there is much work needed to ensure that measures of comparability and quality *do* exist and are adhered to by all organisations. Until that time, qualitative analysis at a national level will always suffer from the sort of criticisms that have been levied to date. Such criticism should ensure that the situation will improve, as only through the analysis of data collected will that data improve.

It should also be borne in mind that the criteria used for extracting data can have as much of an impact on the final reports as the quality of the underlying data. Ensuring that the correct criteria are used is about ensuring that requests for information are specified and interpreted correctly. This is a classic example of the role to be undertaken by an experienced analyst, and, as there is a dearth of such skills within the NHS, misinterpreting requests for information is commonplace.

Given all of this, there should be little wonder that there is such scepticism whenever 'another' IM&T strategy comes along. It is no surprise that there is a view within the NHS and its hierarchy that over the past nine years little progress has been made in terms of delivering robust, qualitative information from existing systems. What is going to change in order to deliver the information required by the groups identified within the latest strategic documents?

The thrust of any IM&T strategy should be about delivering the required information to the required users in the most efficient manner. Previous strategies may not have focused on the information aspects in enough detail because qualitative information has not traditionally been a major agenda item for the NHS. Satisfying the information needs of any group of users should not be too difficult, as long as two very basic prerequisites have been satisfied:

▶ Information requirements have been specified clearly.

▶ The data required to satisfy the information requirements are being collected.

The fundamental prerequisite is, of course, the former: specifying the requirements. The size of this task should not be underestimated.

The vast majority of requests for information are reactive. Pro-active specification of information requirements, designed to assist the monitoring and decision-making processes, is an important way forward and will require significant cultural change.

References

1   NHS Executive. *Information for Health. An Information Strategy for the Modern NHS 1998–2005*. London, 1998.
2   The Welsh Office. *Better Information – Better Health. Information Management and Technology for Health Care and Health Improvement in Wales*. Issued 19 March 1999, Cardiff.
3   *Tabular List of the Classification of Surgical Operations and Procedures, Fourth Revision*. Office of Population Censuses and Surveys, 1990.
4   World Health Organisation. *International Statistical Classification of Diseases and Related Health Problems*, Tenth Revision. Geneva, 1992.
5   NHS Executive. *Clinical Coding Manual*. London, 1994.
6   Adams D. *The Hitch Hiker's Guide to the Galaxy*. London: Pan Books Ltd., 1979.
7   NHS Executive. *Working Together with Health Information. A Partnership Strategy for Education, Training and Development*. London, December 1999.

►10

Clinical Governance in Primary Care. Developing a Strategy for Primary Care Groups

Kieran Sweeney

The origin of clinical governance is unmistakably political. History will show that its roots can be traced back to the election of the Labour administration in May 1997. The incoming government had pledged to abolish the internal market, correct inequalities in provision (the so-called 'post code prescribing issue') and to engage the public more productively in the debate about the planning and delivery of services.

'Policies,' the new government said, 'will build on professional traditions of standard setting and self-regulation.'[1] But in reality, their reforms were an abreaction against the previous administration's programme for the NHS, led by the then Prime Minister Margaret Thatcher. The new government thought the public remained uneasy about an internal market within a publicly funded service; the costs needed to support that system were huge; and quality issues were very rarely addressed despite an explicit contracting system.[2] Quality was to become the central issue. A statutory duty to improve quality at every locality level was introduced. It was given the name 'clinical governance'.

For those in primary care, this was a sea change. At that time, little systematic work had been done to evaluate quality markers in primary care.[3] The fragmented community of the independent contractor general practitioners, together with their evolving relationship with host Health Authorities – not employed but increasingly managed – worked against the adoption of quality improvement programmes. 'Clinical governance' was the buzz phrase, but what exactly did it mean? Scally and Donaldson[4] led the way with a woolly attempt. 'Clinical governance,' they wrote, 'is a system through which NHS organisations are accountable for continuously improving the quality of their services and safeguarding standards of care by creating an environment in which excellence flourishes.' Nobody did or has explained how to create an environment. Individual accountability formed the basis of Professor Pietroni's definition later the same year:[5] 'Clinical governance is the means by which organisations ensure the provision of quality clinical care by making individuals accountable for setting, maintaining and monitoring performance standards.' However it was to be defined, all the commentators on health policy agreed that to succeed, clinical governance would require new ways of working right across organisations, skilled leadership, and a positive culture *shift* in the NHS. For GPs, however, the key issue was poor performance.

So how did clinical governance develop in primary care? In this chapter we recount the experience of clinical governance in one primary care group (PCG) in the south-west of England. What principles guided the development of a quality agenda? What structures were set up to facilitate that process, and to what effect? What specific activities defined the emerging properties of clinical governance, and how were they received? By recounting this experience, we give an honest account of what happened, how it was received, what went well and what went badly, in the hope that others might learn from the experience.

The components of clinical governance

Two principles guided the development of a clinical governance (CG) strategy in the authors' PCG. The first was to pursue lines of work which, if completed, could clearly be expected to improve the clinical care of patients, to relieve their suffering, or to improve their health. The second was to endorse the responsibility of healthcare professionals to use the model of evidence-based practice always but only when it is appropriate.[6] The CG team took a postmodern approach[7] in which the PCG could be regarded as an emerging complex organisation.[8] We think that it is important to be explicit individually and as an organisation about the nature of this approach, as it defines much of what was planned, and because it carried two key implications. First, it is accepted within such an approach that small changes could produce large effects, and *vice versa*: unexpected changes or sudden deviations from tightly crafted plans were not just likely but were guaranteed. Only their type and direction remained uncertain. Second, within this model, the transfer of information occurred in a non-linear way, through loops, reinforcements and interactions with the social and political context within which the NHS was developing.[9] Thus, to assume a linear model, say, for the implementation of good practice would be naïve; to assume that illness was simply biomedical dysfunction, too simple.

Exploring how culture interacted with disease to produce the illness experience – and trying to modify that interaction – was to be the overarching challenge for the PCG.[10] Allen's[11] dictum summed up our position: 'Data can become information if we know the process involved. Information can become knowledge if we know the system that is operating. But knowledge can only become wisdom when we can see how any system must change and can deal with that reality.'

We took Scally and Donaldson's[4] description of CG, adopted their six themes, and developed a series of working principles around them. In the rest of this chapter, we recount how we translated the general principles of clinical governance into specific activities, and describe how these were received by our constituents. These themes and mechanisms are shown in Figure 10.1.

Collaboration

The authors' CG team developed a policy of collaboration with the major stakeholders in the health community, namely the PCG board, the public, the primary care health professional community, and social services. The purpose of developing these alliances was, respectively, to facilitate the implementation of the health improvement

Themes	Working principles
Collaboration	▶ Health Improvement Programme (HIMP)
	▶ Practice clinical governance leads meetings
	▶ Work on involving the public
	▶ Develop relationships with social services
Risk avoidance	▶ Learning from complaints and mistakes
	▶ Regular review of practice systems
	▶ Develop occupational health service
Poor performance	▶ Develop procedures for reporting concerns early
	▶ Significant event audit meetings
	▶ Encourage nurse clinical supervision
Quality methods	▶ Evidence-based practice
	▶ Educational plans
	▶ Develop audit programme
Culture	▶ Work on citizen involvement
	▶ Developing leadership
	▶ Bottom-up change in thinking
Infrastructure	▶ Secure proper funding
	▶ Develop formal clinical governance teamwork and business meetings
	▶ Work in information and technology departments
	▶ Develop a system of securing good quality primary care clinical data

Figure 10.1. Clinical governance themes

programme (HIMP), to encourage a climate of transparency and accountability to the local citizens, to foster a corporate feel to the fragmented community of twenty general practices within the PCG, and to recognise the importance of creating joint responsibility for prioritising and funding services that straddled the unhelpful and artefactual health/social divide. It looked good in theory; so how did it work in practice?

The clinical governance team identified three national priority areas which would form part of the HIMP – coronary heart disease, mental illness and cancer – and set about engaging with practices and key players to develop a relevant programme of work for each area. For heart disease, the team set up a half-day meeting with representatives of all practices in the city, at which all practices agreed to formulate a protocol for the care of patients with ischaemic heart disease, and lodge it with the clinical governance team. The team had hoped to secure agreement with all practices on the precise terms for recording key cardiac diagnoses, which would form the basis of a grounded prevalence database. This proved more difficult than expected and work continues on the data-recording mechanisms. The diagnosis and management of dementia provided a forum for further collaboration with the PCG and selected representatives of social services. The CG team formed part of a long-term service agreement working party, which developed a multidisciplinary approach to the topic. The group worked in collaboration with the audit department within the Health Authority, who were developing a new set of evidence-based guidelines in consultation with primary and secondary care, as well as social services and psychologists.

The highly publicised trial of the mass murderer Dr Harold Shipman shook the public's confidence in the medical profession, and clearly demanded a fresh and vigorous strategy for involving the public. At the macro level, the PCG board convened a public meeting at which the local health policy and CG strategy was set out, questioned and criticised. But consulting the public went beyond such meetings: individual practices served the public in the form of their registered population, and nurses and doctors served the public too in each consultation they held. To address the former, practices were encouraged to form patient liaison or participation groups, and those with expertise in the area invited to share their experience. In consultations, the interpersonal skills of the professionals were central. How could the public comment on these skills? The authors' CG team looked to the Australian Royal College of General Practitioners for their example. There, public involvement had become one of the criteria for re-certification of doctors, a questionnaire had been developed for the purpose, and a substantial body of literature describing its validation and impact published.[12] All the practices in our PCG agreed to distribute the questionnaire to around 2500 patients.

At the time of writing, the results are being analysed and fed back to the participating professionals, who have, in turn, been invited to share their aggregated practice data with the CG team, to form part of the PCG report at the end of the year. Figure 10.2 links the working principles of collaboration outlined in Figure 10.1 with the specific activities described above.

Risk avoidance

Risk avoidance means learning from mistakes (or near misses) and reviewing the adequacy of practice clinical and organisational safety systems. Ensuring and preserving the good health of primary care team members counts also. A central plank

Working principles	Specific activity
Health Improvement Programme	▶ Identify key clinical areas with PCG board, convene meeting with constituent practices to work on protocols and data collection in these areas
Practice clinical governance leads meetings	▶ Funded by the PCG to cover locum costs. These meetings created a networking forum for practices and an opportunity to set out CG policy
Involving the public	▶ Macro level: public meeting
	▶ Micro level: distribution of interpersonal skills questionnaire
Involving Social Services	▶ Collaboration in working party for long-term service agreement for dementia management

Figure 10.2. Collaboration: turning theory into practice

of this part of the policy was to encourage regular significant event audit (SEA) meetings whose relevance to the development of general practice was just being recognised at that time.[13] A capability and capacity survey early in the first year of the PCG showed that most practices in the city were holding regular SEA meetings, documenting their results and reviewing them periodically. Continuing liaison with the local audit group ensured that appropriate training meetings were made available to practices not actively involved in SEA.

By the end of the first year, all practices were doing SEA or had been trained for it. Inhouse complaints systems were reviewed by the team members during the practice visits, and particular attention was paid to how they were documented, and how the practice learned from them.

Recognising that maintaining the health of team members, while desirable in itself, also was a part of a comprehensive risk management strategy is fairly new to primary care. Personnel employed in hospitals and Health Authorities enjoyed comprehensive occupational health services (OHSs). That those in general practice did not was an anachronism that had to be addressed. The CG team constructed a full business case to put to the board, whose agreement with the proposal was underwritten with full funding (of around £12 500) for one year. A full evaluation of the programme was written into the bid, which will continue to attract funding as and when evidence of its value is collected.

Poor performance

The public were in no doubt that they needed protection from underperforming doctors and were aghast at the perceived reluctance of the medical profession to grasp

Working principle	Specific activity
Learning from complaints and mistakes	▶ Assess how many practices were carrying out SEA, and encourage all practices to participate in SEA
Regular review of practice systems	▶ Direct evaluation of in house complaints systems during practice visits
Develop occupational health service (OHS)	▶ Put business case, secure funding, build in evaluation, and make service available OHS to all practices

Figure 10.3.   Risk management: turning theory into practice

the nettle. The debacles in breast screening in Exeter, and heart surgery in Bristol, concentrated the mind on the task, and Dr Shipman's mass murders rendered professional sensitivity an historical luxury. Things had to change; systems to secure the core confidence of the public set in place quickly.

The authors' CG team supported the General Medical Council's principle of self-regulation, an idea under siege, but clearly a powerful engine for change in the right circumstances.[14] But the government was unimpressed: their publication *Supporting Doctors; Protecting Patients*[15] proposed annual appraisal for doctors and regional support centres for failing doctors. While the details of this astonishing document were awaited, the joint publication of the General Practice Committee of the British Medical Association and the Royal College of General Practitioners, *Good Medical Practice for General Practitioners*,[16] describing unacceptable and excellent performance, formed the bedrock of the authors' PCG policy. Closer collaboration with the local medical committee (LMC), who had considerable experience in this area, was planned. The role of SEA in identifying areas where performance might be improved was stressed. For nurses, clinical supervision was gaining in popularity and momentum, even if evidence of its effectiveness was slim. Ill health is often a contributing factor in poor performance, so having access to an OHS locally was welcomed.

Quality methods

The six themes of CG chosen as the scaffolding for the quality agenda clearly overlap with each other. The quality agenda developed by the authors' CG team in collaboration with the PCG included many of the elements mentioned above – SEA, protocol development and clinical supervision, for example. The work on the long-term service agreement for a multidisciplinary dementia service, and evaluation of the innovative walk-in centre and primary care service for the homeless were additional strands in the quality thread. But education formed the nub of the quality approach, in the form of PCG-wide educational study days. These were multidisciplinary, involved

Working principle	Specific activity
Developing procedures for reporting concerns early	▶ Collaborate with LMC, and use their experience
	▶ Develop a local written policy for poor performance based on national professional bodies' guidance, in collaboration with Health Authority
	▶ Collaborate with the local OHS to develop their contribution in this area
SEA meetings	▶ Encourage these and focus on issues of improving performance
Nurse clinical supervision	▶ Promote, and try to collate evidence of effectiveness

Figure 10.4. Poor performance: turning theory into practice

representatives of every constituent practice, and presented a programme comprising a keynote address with supporting parallel sessions preselected by the delegates. Practices were provided with funds to cover locum costs. The keynote topics included guideline development and occupational health. In supporting workshops, delegates chose between involving the public, communication, continuing professional development, personal learning plans, direct nurse access in general practice, working with social services, SEA and appraisals. Delegates, judging from their feedback, derived as much benefit from their interaction with other practices as from the sessions themselves. This was clearly an opportunity to develop a true corporate feel in the PCG, which began to turn the rhetoric of collaboration into reality.

An increasing number of retained, non-principal, locum and itinerant doctors worked outside this mainstream of health professionals, however, and public confidence in their competence had to be secured, as far as possible using conventional professional standards. At that time, retained doctors remained supported only through the Deanery arrangements, which often were relatively unresponsive to local circumstances. Locum doctors had little formal association with CG either. The team drew up a plan of gradual integration of these two groups, as well as the doctors serving the local prison. Figure 10.5 summarises the quality agenda and activities for this.

Culture

In theory, accountability is the cornerstone of clinical governance. In practice, this means two things: it means being professionally accountable through revalidation, external audit, and continuing professional development; but more than that, it means

Working principles	Specific activity
Evidence-based practice	▶ Encourage evidence-based practice in dementia service and through protocol development
Educational plans	▶ Study days organised for all practices and funded through the PCG
Audit programme	▶ Identify programme of audits that related to the topics identified in the HIMP, and arising out of SEA

Figure 10.5. Quality agenda: turning theory into practice

being accountable to the public too – at the population, local or individual level. Consulting the public, genuinely involving them in the health debate, and seeking their views on professional performance thus becomes an additional part of clinical governance. Few would risk arguing against such principles, but how to do it?

The authors' CG team devised a three-pronged strategy. The first two components – patient participation groups in practices and the distribution of the interpersonal skills questionnaire – have been described earlier. But there still remained the problem of ensuring that public representatives could engage in the sometimes esoteric debate about local and national health issues. Understanding even the terms of such a debate could be difficult – comparing standardised mortality ratios, or appraising the evidence for a new technology, for example. The CG team collaborated with the local research and development support unit (RDSU) to secure funds to devise and present a series of workshops for lay members of PCGs, Health Authorities and Trusts. The workshops will run throughout the autumn of 2000, with a simultaneous programme of evaluation to ensure the workshops can be refined and improved.

This programme of public accountability demanded resources and manpower beyond the capacity of the appointed CG team. Throughout their first year, the CG team identified local leaders from practices, audit groups and the Health Authority, who could participate at key points in the programme, for example by presenting on particular topics with which they had special knowledge (such as personal development plans) or disseminating skills (for example, information technology). 'Bottom-up thinking' is a buzz phrase of the moment, implying the desirable aim of incorporating frontline thinking into policy. But how to do it? Throughout the first year of their work, the CG team visited every constituent practice, recording their views on how CG should develop, noting any concerns about the practice activity, and feeding back into the PCG good ideas about day to day working.

Small practices expressed problems in providing members to attend meetings or serve on committees; large practices felt disadvantaged by attempts to achieve financial equity between practices where their economies of scale on staff and equipment were not rewarded. One practice had a highly developed service offering alternative therapies once a week. Another had pioneered direct access to nurses for acute, minor illness. These activities are summarised in Figure 10.6.

Working principles	Specific activity
Working on citizen involvement	▶ Develop patient participation groups
	▶ Disseminate interpersonal skills questionnaire
	▶ Devise workshops to facilitate lay member involvement at PCG or board level
Leadership	▶ Spotting and recruiting local leaders with particular skills to participate at key points in the programme
Bottom up thinking	▶ Practice visits to constituents, feedback of good ideas

Figure 10.6.   Changing culture: turning theory into practice

Infrastructure

None of the clinical governance work can proceed without proper resources, protected time and adequate infrastructure. While there is anecdotal evidence of great variability in the rate of remuneration of clinical governance leads, far-sighted chief executives in Health Authorities secured suitable funding (equivalent to consultant rates) and enough protected time for the leads (in the authors' case, two days per week, shared between two joint leads). A support officer, good computers, secretarial support and access to electronic search facilities provided an agreeable backdrop for the work to proceed. A CG subcommittee was convened, met every two months, recorded minutes, and delegated tasks to its membership, which was drawn from primary care in the broadest sense: a dentist, pharmacist, social worker and lay person sat alongside the nurse, audit person, PAM (professions allied to medicine) representative and two doctors.

The need to upgrade computer facilities in the constituent practices was spotted in the early days of the CG team's work. A capability and capacity stock take was undertaken across all PCGs in the autumn of 1999, which had revealed wide variations in equipment, gaps in IT skills and different training needs across the practices. The CG team distinguished between the operational side of IT – the remit of the commercial companies – and a separate quality dimension to IT, which was within the team's terms of reference. The ability to manage and display clinical data well, and to share data across practices and ultimately between PCGs, was seen as a legitimate aspiration for the team. Together with clinical governance links in practices, the CG leads agreed to lead on the development of a minimum data set for patients, to be recorded on computer, and subsequently shared.

The authors secured funding for an 'AA' man (ie 'I know a man who can') for computer maintenance and development within the PCG. A small additional sum was allocated to develop a portfolio of equipment for practices under three headings – essential, desirable and luxurious – from which practices made bids. In this way, the

Working principle	Specific activity
Secure funding	► Consultant rates for doctors, two days per week shared between joint leads
Develop formal subcommittee	► Convened, minutes recorded, tasks delegated
Improve computer skills and facilities	► 'AA' man in post. Small fund for improving computer/clinical facilities
Improve primary care clinical data	► Agree minimum data set

Figure 10.7.   Infrastructure: turning rhetoric into reality

CG team felt able to improve the availability of top class clinical equipment for patients in their locality. Figure 10.7 summarises this part of the team's work.

Summary

Is any of this going to make a difference? And what are the best ways of recognising any emerging benefits from the approach that the authors describe? Clearly a discernible decrease in morbidity and mortality in target conditions in the priority areas included in the PCG's HIMP would be the gold standard outcome, but the time taken for these differences to become clear and problems of attribution might make this an elusive measurement. A robust database of the key conditions of interest to the PCG (as part of their HIMP, or their responsibility for national frameworks) is more easily secured and monitored; this could be viewed as a proxy marker for more direct benefit. Greater involvement of public health specialists in CG work will facilitate this and will constitute another marker of successful implementation of this CG strategy. The longer-term success of this developing CG strategy should be judged by the imminent requirement for revalidation of doctors. The whole CG policy should be moulded around this, so that when it comes, many of the standards are already in place, are being monitored and are up to standard in all practices. 2001 sees the start of the first round of evaluations by the Commission for Health Improvement (CHI). The CG team will ensure, as far as it can, that its activities are compatible with the requirements of this statutory body; so that its assessment – which will be searching, and conducted very much in the public gaze – will be met using quality markers that are part of day to day quality general practice, and not invented specially for the purpose. Patients remain at the centre of any approach; ensuring their productive (and not just nominal) involvement at board level, continuing to record their views on services through serial distribution of the improving practice questionnaire, and seeking other ways of involving them in the health debate will continue to be central planks of clinical governance policy for this PCG. At a time when the culture of the NHS is changing faster than ever, there is no time for complacency. *Carpe diem*!

References

1   Shapiro J. The new NHS: commentaries on the White paper: encouraging responsibility, different pathways to accountability. *BMJ* 1998; 316: 296–297.

2   Gray JD, Donaldson LJ. Improving the quality of health care through contracting; a study of health authority practice. *Quality in Health Care* 1996; 5: 201–205.

3   Marshall M. Conference presentation: National Association University Departments of General Practice, Bournmouth, July 2000.

4   Scally F, Donaldson L. Clinical governance and the drive for quality improvement in the new NHS in England. *BMJ* 1998; 317: 61–63.

5   Pietroni P. Clinical governance in primary care groups. Address to clinical governance leads, RHA Conference, Dillington House, November 1998.

6   Sweeney KG. The information paradox. In: M Marinker (ed.) *Sense and Sensibility in Health Care.* London: BMJ Publishing Group, 1996: 59–87.

7   Gray JAM. Postmodern medicine. *Lancet* 1999; 354: 1550–1553.

8   Funcowicz S, Revetz J. Emergent complex systems. *Futures* 1994; 26(6): 568–582.

9   Cillers P. *Complexity and Postmodernism.* London/New York: Routledge, 1998.

10 Morris P. *Illness and Culture in the Postmodern Age.* San Francisco: University of California Press, 1998.

11 Allen PM. Coherence chaos and evolution in the social context. *Futures* 1994; 26(6): 583–597.

12 Greco M, Cavanagh M, Brownlea A, McGovern J. The Doctor Interpersonal Skills Questionnaire (DISQ): a validated instrument for use in GP training. *Education for General Practice* 1999; 10: 256–264.

13 Westcott R, Sweeney G, Stead J. Significant event auditing in practice: a preliminary study. *Family Practice* 2000; 17(2): 173–179.

14 Hamilton W, Bradley N. Self-regulation at work: a case study. *BMJ* 1999; 319: 585.

15 Department of Health. *Supporting Doctors; Protecting Patients.* London: The Stationery Office, 1999.

16 General Practice Committee of the British Medical Association and the Royal College of General Practitioners. *Good Medical Practice for General Practitioners.* London, 2000.

▶11

NICE and Clinical Governance

Andrew Dillon

The medium and the message

Just after the National Institute for Clinical Excellence (NICE) was formed, *The Economist* commented that the new organisation was '... at the forefront of international health-care reform'.[1] This rather flattering observation was appropriately contextualised with a description of the other mechanisms that the NHS was, at that time, beginning to introduce – including, of course, clinical governance. No one with any knowledge of the processes involved in getting research into practice would have needed to be told that however carefully crafted the guidance produced by the Institute, it would need an implementation vehicle to secure its proper influence in clinical practice. This vehicle is clinical governance.

Similarly, if the central purpose of clinical governance is to secure for patients a consistently high quality of clinical care, those responsible for operating it will need to have measurable standards to which to work. Accessing opinion on what might constitute desirable standards in any aspect of medicine is very easy; deciding what to select as the preferred definition of best practice is more difficult. There are, for example, 24 guidelines on asthma cited on Medline, even using a very narrowly defined search strategy.[2] Even if a single NHS organisation (or even a whole local health economy) could agree on a single option, the likelihood of the NHS as a whole simultaneously arriving at the same conclusion is remote. Considered in the context of this ocean of advice, the case for national guidance, produced from a single authoritative source, becomes compelling. With NICE, clinical governance has been given an important part of its payload.

The Institute and its contribution

NICE was established in April 1999, to provide guidance to patients and health professionals in England and Wales on the clinical and cost effectiveness of selected technologies and other health interventions. The Institute does this through undertaking health technology appraisals, commissioning clinical guidelines, and funding clinical audit at a national level. NICE also provides funding for a range of effective practice publications.

The Institute is a Special Health Authority, placing it firmly inside the National Health Service. It is a small organisation, employing around 28 people (on June 2000). It commissions much of the research underpinning its guidance from other organisations and groups, both inside and outside the NHS, which provides it with considerable strength in depth, by developing partnerships with centres of academic excellence and the national professional bodies. Its approach to its work is transparent and inclusive, designed to generate confidence in the objectivity of its approach and ownership of its guidance.

The Institute is part of a process of modernisation of the NHS in England and Wales. There are a number of new and existing bodies, such as the Commission for Health Improvement (CHI), the Health Development Agency (HDA) and the NHS Research and Development (R&D) Programme, which together aim to improve the quality of clinical practice and service delivery. The Institute shares the view that it is important that these organisations work together effectively to make more for the NHS than just the sum of their parts. These organisations have the ability to support the people who rely on the NHS for their care and those who provide that care, by setting standards and by helping the NHS to assess its performance against those standards, and, when necessary, to improve that performance. They also have the capacity to make life more difficult, however, by failing to manage their boundaries, leaving important gaps, and by ignoring opportunities to eliminate duplication or publishing related products without thinking about how the NHS will have to action them. The advent of NICE should address these problems. The Institute also works closely with the agencies in Scotland that perform similar functions as the CHI, HDA and the NHS R&D Programme in England and Wales, including the Scottish Intercollegiate Guidelines Network (SIGN) and the Health Technology Assessment Board for Scotland (HTB).

So, having close working relationships is important; for example, the Institute needs to share its approach to implementation advice with the CHI. Trusts, primary care groups (PCGs), local health groups (LHGs) and Health Authorities will want to feel secure that where they have followed the Institute's advice on the management of a clinical condition or in the use of a technology, the Commission will accept that approach. Similarly, the Audit Commission's work on best value in the delivery of services needs to dovetail with any guidelines produced by the Institute for related clinical practice. Here, it will be important to avoid any duplication and to ensure complimentary advice. Similarly, the Institute is coordinating carefully its programme of work with the NHS R&D Programme, which will continue to undertake health technology assessments, but over a much longer time scale than the relatively rapid reviews undertaken by NICE. Some of these assessments will be used by the Institute as the basis of its appraisals, effectively providing a 'front end' to the R&D Programme's work.

Technology appraisals include those for pharmaceuticals, medical devices, diagnostic procedures and equipment, clinical procedures and certain aspects of health promotion. Topics are selected for the Institute by the Department of Health in England and by the National Assembly for Wales, following consultation with stakeholders in the process – inside and outside the NHS – against a reference framework formed by the priorities set for the NHS and the emerging National Service Frameworks (NSFs).

The Institute commissions systematic reviews of the clinical and cost effectiveness of technologies from university departments. These reviews, which typically take around 12 months to complete, rely on data in the public domain and that supplied by manufacturers. By 2001, the Institute will be producing, on average, four sets of technology guidelines each month. Clinical guidelines will be commissioned from multidisciplinary authoring groups. Like the technology appraisals, they will be based on a rigorous review of the evidence, taking into account both clinical- and cost-effectiveness. These guidelines will take between 12 and 24 months to complete. The Institute plans to produce between 12 and 15 guidelines each year (possibly more, as the programme develops), supplemented by the guidelines delivered through the PRODIGY primary care decision support system. The authoring of guidance in PRODIGY is the Institute's responsibility, although the software architecture remains with the Department of Health. This programme represents a substantial workload for a young organisation, requiring close planning and careful quality control.

The Institute draws together a range of national clinical audit responsibilities. These responsibilities cover full national multidisciplinary audits, undertaken by consortia of professional groups, and those for funding and controlling the overall direction of the four national Confidential Enquiries. The Institute also funds the *Effectiveness Series,* produced by the Centre for Reviews and Dissemination at York University. These guidelines and technology appraisals will be brought together with clinical audits and audit methodologies as integrated packages of guidance.

NICE's challenge is to bring together these guidance authoring and audit responsibilities in ways which will leverage maximum incremental improvement in the quality of care available through the NHS. In doing so, NICE will help to populate the evidence landscape on which clinical governance relies.

The need for national guidance

It could reasonably be argued that this evidence landscape is already overpopulated. Clinicians and managers already have a wealth of information to select from to inform their standard-setting. So, what is the case for a single statement of best practice from NICE? In summary, the benefits can be stated as follows:

- There is a consistent definition of best practice.
- There is economy of effort from a single, thorough appraisal of the evidence.
- Health professionals and patients can be informed simultaneously.
- There is equitable access to clinical services.
- There is consistent use of resources.

The most widely advertised reason for the creation of NICE is the contribution that an authoritative statement for best practice can make to removing at least the most obvious examples of 'post code prescribing'. Geographical variations in both the quality of clinical practice and in access to technologies have probably always existed in the NHS. However, the very public arrangements for funding services, which developed as part of the reforms introduced in 1990,[3] brought such variations into much sharper focus. Arrangements for funding expensive new technologies and even individual treatments often were the subject of public, and sometimes acrimonious, debate. The case of 'Child B' in Cambridge, in which the local Health Authority refused to fund treatment,[4] and the significant variation in the availability of funding for taxanes in the treatment of breast and ovarian cancer,[5] are just two examples. The view of the government up to the mid-1990s was, generally, that local Health Authorities were responsible, in conjunction with their providers, for deciding how resources should be applied, other than in circumstances where the government had made a determination at a national level.

This forced local health economies to assess and then decide on the merits of new and existing technologies themselves. In some cases, the cost of the technology was the single determinant. In others, attempts were made to appraise the clinical and cost effectiveness of the technology. In some cases, local Trusts and Health Authorities based their decisions on the clinical guidelines developed by the national professional organisations. This has led to a patchwork of access that is defensible neither at local nor national level.

Oddly, perhaps, given the normal remedy offered for solving NHS problems, increasing resources (as occurred in April 2000, with the announcement of a substantial increase in NHS resources) is not, by itself, the solution. Without a single, thorough appraisal of the evidence, geographical variations will continue, since it is unlikely that precisely similar decisions will be taken in the case of every significant technology. This is because, in many cases, determination of the significance of the incremental benefit to patients offered by the technology under scrutiny and its cost effectiveness in a cash-limited service is a matter of judgement, rather than calculation.

It seems a reasonable hypothesis that if an agreed mechanism can be found for determining at a national level the significant aspects of clinical practice, which has the confidence of health professionals and patients, the process itself, at least, will be efficient. This is because it will avoid the need for multiple, often simultaneous interrogation of the same evidence base and the consequent waste of resources (including those of the manufacturers, who often face multiple applications for the same data). A single process can have built into it suitable safeguards for the various stakeholders, and is likely to achieve a high degree of consistency in both methodology and outcome.

Once the guidance has been formulated, it can be disseminated rapidly to health professionals and the public. By using communication vehicles in professional and patient organisations, as well as through NHS management messaging, precisely the same information can be communicated at the same time. Patients will receive the same care on the same basis across the service, which will have had a clear steer on the application of its resources.

So, is there a downside to the development of a programme of national guidance? It might be argued that unless every aspect of the way in which Health Authorities apply their funds (and for that matter, every aspect of the way in which clinicians practice) is the subject of national guidance – whatever the benefits to the patients who gain from national guidance – the process of local priority-setting will be distorted. Even with clear national priorities and NSFs, different populations will present different demands for service. NICE guidance, it might be said, takes something away from the important dialogue between local health organisations and the people who rely on them for their care, by avoiding the need for those organisations to involve the local population in a dialogue about how to apply devolved funds.

Each local health economy has its priorities. Many of these will coincide with NICE guidance because Health Authorities and Trusts will want to ensure that they are funding clinically and cost effective practice in mainstream service areas. But what about those local priorities that NICE guidance does not cover? It is clear that the Institute's guidance will remove some discretion from local health organisations. But in all cases, it will be to direct funds into areas in which those organisations will inevitably have to spend money anyway. Our guidance will ensure that it is spent effectively.

Does nationally determined guidance remove or compromise clinical freedom? To answer this, we should ask what is meant by 'clinical freedom'. One definition might be that it is a form of permission in which patients allow clinicians to treat them as part of an unwritten contract. Such permission assumes that the patient will have access to:

▶ a competent clinical practitioner

▶ dialogue with their practitioner

▶ the diagnosis

▶ options for treatment

▶ treatment selected on the basis of the evidence of what works.

Given that NICE is about providing information to patients and health professionals on what works, far from *limiting* clinical freedom (at least on the basis of this definition), it actually *informs* it.

Contributing to clinical governance

One approach to clinical governance requires the leaders of NHS organisation to ask the following questions: What do we expect of ourselves? What tests are we going to apply to our performance from which we can draw conclusions about the quality of what we do? Which benchmarks adequately describe our definition of a good standard of care. And perhaps the most searching of all questions: What would we expect for ourselves as patients using our own services?

Locally developed standards have the advantage – in theory at least – of the prospect of good local ownership and therefore implementation. Development is likely to be inclusive, stimulating the involvement of those whom will need to weave them into their own day-to-day clinical practice. They can be tested as they are developed, at a very personal level. A further advantage is that the topics will, by definition, be those of immediate relevance to the health professionals and managers using them. Getting local ownership is a real challenge for those responsible for authoring guidance at a national level. It is part of the wider issue of implementation.

Whilst it is likely that the Institute's guidance will be given considerable exposure, through the clinical governance systems in place in Trusts, PCGs and LHGs, the fact that it is NICE guidance will not, of itself, be enough to secure implementation. This is particularly true of the clinical guidelines programme. The question for NICE – and those working with the Institute in developing its guidance (particularly clinical guidelines) – is, what can be done by the Institute to help secure the comprehensive implementation of its guidance? Broadly, the Institute's contribution is likely to be through:

▶ topic selection

▶ an inclusive and transparent authoring process

▶ presentation of the guidance

▶ effective dissemination

▶ practical implementation advice

▶ an audit methodology for both process and outcomes, and

▶ regular review of the guidance.

Topic selection

The Institute is commissioned to undertake technology appraisals and to prepare clinical guidelines by the Department of Health and the National Assembly for Wales. The framework is set by the priorities that have been selected for the NHS and the NSFs. The authors of the NSFs identify technologies, guidelines and audits with which they wish to populate each Framework. These topics are fed into the Managing Clinical Interventions Group (MCIG), a joint committee of the Department of Health (DoH) and the National Assembly for Wales (NAW). MCIG is made up of policy leads from the Department and the Assembly and others from Regional Offices in England. The Group receives reports from the Horizon Scanning Centre at the University of Birmingham, and searches information in the public domain for significant new technologies likely to meet the criteria for selection of topics for NICE. MCIG also takes account of the output of the NHS R&D Programme. The criteria used to select topics for the Institute's work programmes are as follows:[6]

i) Overall significance to the NHS
The appraisal process is intended as much to promote the faster dissemination of products likely to achieve worthwhile health gain as it is to discourage the dissemination of products that are not clinically cost effective.

ii) Significant management challenge in effective introduction of the intervention
Some innovations, however desirable in principle, nevertheless may require careful attention by NHS management if they are to be introduced successfully. This is not just a question of securing financial resources; the potential impact on other NHS resources requires consideration.

iii) Likelihood of significant misallocation of resources in the absence of guidelines
Other things being equal, guidance will be more valuable if it 'adds value' – in other words, if it encourages clinicians and patients to make more informed decisions than they would have done unaided. Examples are as follows:

▶ Treatments for life-threatening or disabling conditions for which no good treatment yet exists.

▶ Treatments where the most readily measurable clinical endpoints do not easily translate into measures of patient wellbeing.

▶ Treatments over which there might be serious ethical concerns.

▶ Treatments where there is serious doubt as to whether they are appropriate for NHS funding for the generality of patients.

▶ Existing treatments where there is controversy over best practice or where there is evidence of significant departures from best practice.

The importance of engaging the NHS in setting the Institute's agenda is recognised, and in England, Regional Offices are consulted on what are considered to be the most significant issues. Wales has separate arrangements for informing its judgements on priority topics. Whether this process of consultation with the service is sufficient to secure the local ownership that will be crucial for effective implementation remains to be seen. It is likely that demand from the service will lead to a broader engagement over time.

Inclusive and transparent appraisal and authoring processes

The arrangements for involving interested parties in appraising technologies have been in place since the autumn of 1999. Relevant national professional (including NHS management) and patient organisations are identified, alongside the commercial sponsors for manufactured technologies. The Appraisal Committee has the ability to invite clinicians and patient advocates to inform its consideration of individual technologies, and it has begun to do so. The appraisal process (shown in Figure 11.1) allows for these groups to submit evidence and to comment on the emerging guidance at two stages, before it is released to the NHS. Wider and more open engagement with NHS professionals and patients would be possible using the Internet, but it is doubtful that the Appraisal Committee would be able, usefully, to take such unstructured comment into account in the time allocated to its consideration of each technology.

An interesting tension arises here, between the desire for involvement and transparency and the need – perceived particularly by the manufacturers – for confidentiality. Some information submitted is commercially confidential. In certain circumstances, such information might be share-price sensitive and its deliberate misuse is a criminal offence. In practice, whilst the Institute can ensure that

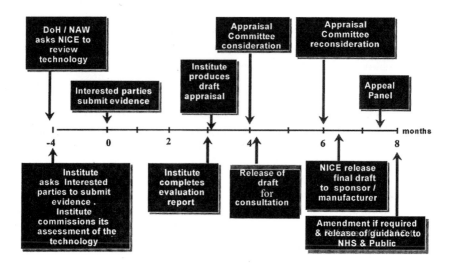

Fig. 11.1. Diagrammatic representation of appraisal process. DoH, Department of Health; NAW, National Assembly of Wales

commercially sensitive data is held securely, once the process of consultation on the emerging guidance begins (which draws on, but does not actually disclose, commercially confidential information), involving, as it does, many groups, it is very difficult to avoid the direction of the Committee's thinking finding its way into the public domain.

The process for producing clinical guidelines is broadly similar. Although neither the Institute nor its Guidelines Advisory Committee actually writes the guidelines, the principles of inclusion and transparency apply in the same way. National groups are consulted and the emerging guideline is exposed to comment as it develops. The guidelines authoring groups will comprise health professionals and patient advocates. Although not full clinical guidelines, the Institute's Referral Guides (advice for general practitioners and their colleagues in primary care in referring patients on to specialist care), published for piloting in June 2000,[7] show how it is possible for a national organisation to connect successfully with practising clinicians. Each of the 11 Guides was developed by a multidisciplinary advisory group which, together, drew in over 50 health professionals.

Presentation of the guidance

The presentation of the guidance also is likely to influence its adoption. It seems reasonable to speculate that clear, concise and definitive documents, with accessible summaries, will encourage use. NICE intends to break new ground in the way its guidance is presented. Its first documents have been well received by the service. Generally, this will mean that a summary will be available for each area of guidance.

For technology appraisals, for example, this occupies less than one side of A4 paper. All guidance will be available online, in portable document format, and it will be engineered into the PRODIGY decision support system used in general practice. The Institute sees electronic presentation as the way forward in presenting guidance to clinicians and managers at the right time and in a useable format. For managers, this might be in an executive information system or on an intranet. For clinicians, we would want our guidance to be available through the software that supports the electronic patient record. We have commissioned a version that can be downloaded into a Psion organiser for completely portable access, and we have entered into agreements for organisations, such as the National Electronic Library for Health, which works with clinicians to present clinical guidelines electronically, to carry the Institute's guidance.

The presentation format we have chosen for our technology appraisal guidance documents is deliberately intended to engage as wide an audience as possible. These documents are short – usually around four or five pages, with appendices – and written in a style likely to be understood by an informed, non-clinical reader. There is a separate 'patient notes' section, written in conjunction with a relevant national patient advocate organisation.

The document is split into nine sections:

1 The guidance itself
2 Clinical need and practice
3 A description of the technology
4 The evidence base for the appraisal
5 The implications of the guidance for the NHS
6 Any further research which the Institute recommends the NHS should encourage
7 Any related Institute guidance
8 Advice on implementation of the guidance by NHS organisations
9 Clinical audit methodology
10 The date on which the Institute will review the guidance.

This gives the reader the basic audit trail from the evidence to the conclusion. More information, including the full Assessment Report used by the Appraisal Committee, is available on the Institute's website (URL: www.nice.org.uk).

Effective dissemination

Some of the approaches that the Institute is taking to disseminate information and, in particular, its intention to use electronic media to get advice to clinicians and mangers, is described above. An equal amount of effort is put into communicating guidance to the public as to ensuring that clinicians and managers are aware of it. This is intended to address both the intention to open up decision-making processes in the NHS and to help to develop the public's ability to act as informed consumers. Clinicians and managers will find that pressure for implementation of NICE guidance will come not just from the NHS but also directly from patients, who will know what they can expect from the NHS in the areas covered by the Institute's guidance. NICE guidance is just as likely to appear in *Womens Own* as it is in the *BMJ*.

Practical implementation advice

One of the challenges laid at the door of the Institute is that its guidance will count for very little unless the NHS can do significantly better than most healthcare systems in securing comprehensive implementation of its advice. It is argued that however effectively we communicate our work, for it to positively influence clinical practice it will have to be woven into the fabric of the daily practice of thousands of clinicians. The question for the Institute is, what is the role for a small national organisation in implementing its guidance? The quality and consistency of what is produced is obviously important, as is the effectiveness of its dissemination. Getting advice on new technologies at the point at which they are introduced also is critical, as is producing the clinical guidelines that will populate NSFs at the point they are launched. The Institute's technology appraisal guidance already contains implementation advice, designed to give it a 'pre-washed' feel. It is written both to help NHS organisations demonstrate compliance and as a test of implementability, before the guidance is actually issued. Clinical guidelines will contain similar advice.

So, whilst our guidance will include general advice on implementation strategies, the Institute has neither the responsibility nor the capacity to act directly in ensuring the implementation of its advice. This is presumed to rest with Health Authorities, Trusts and PCGs. The Institute is concerned that, whilst responsibility for implementation should remain with these bodies, there remains a large potential gap, particularly between the publication of its clinical guidelines and the necessary action required at a local level. Although implementation clearly is essential for its technology appraisal guidance, it is likely that the decision-making process involved in, for example, getting a new drug into a PCG/LHG or hospital formulary will be significantly less complicated than implementing a full clinical guideline on the management of a condition, which could involve health professionals in more than one organisation (and could possibly involve the local Social Services agencies and voluntary organisations). In these circumstances, one solution would be for implementation in each local health economy to be supported and coordinated by a group of health professionals seconded from their routine clinical practice for a specific period. This would have a high up-front cost but it would be time-limited and is likely to have downstream benefit in terms of ownership and impact.

An audit methodology for both process and outcome

Clinicians and the organisations that employ them will want to measure both the effectiveness of their implementation arrangements and how their practice compares with national benchmarks. The Institute's technology appraisal guidance sets out (where appropriate) specific access criteria to enable the precise deployment of an individual technology. Using its network of partnerships with national professional organisations, organised into a series of NICE Collaborating Centres, the Institute will commission specific audits to populate the guidelines, both before and after they are issued.

Regular review of guidance

Both clinicians and managers will want to know that the Institute's guidance will be kept up to date, and ensuring that this happens is critical to the Institute's continuing credibility. Each piece of guidance will be published with a review date. This will act as a long stop, rather than defining the fixed amount of time that will be allowed to elapse before the guidance is updated. The Institute will arrange to scan the evidence landscape periodically, looking for significant new information. When sufficient evidence has accumulated, whenever this occurs, the guidance will be reviewed and if necessary updated. Updates will be available immediately on the Institute's website, and published biannually in the Institute's national guidelines publication.

Conclusions

NHS organisations are finding that much of clinical governance is an evolution of the systems, structures and performance measurement that they already had, to a greater or lesser extent, put in place. The government's focus (and that of the professional organisations) on the active management of the quality of services and of individual performance has placed this task at the top of the NHS agenda. For chief executives and their senior colleagues, while the imperatives to manage the money effectively and to perform against increasingly demanding access criteria are still very much present, it is the quality of the services for which they are responsible which now stands as their key performance indicator. Their personal involvement in these systems and structures is, in effect, mandatory, and this fact on its own has changed the nature of the way in which the standard of clinical practice will be managed in the future.

For most, if not all, NHS organisations, however, it is the change in the culture of the organisation that will be the most demanding challenge. Structures and systems, to the extent they are required, are relatively easy to put in place. In some Trusts, the first action taken when the clinical governance initiative was announced was to establish a Clinical Governance Committee. In others, the initial response was to reflect on what the NHS was being asked to do and to consider how their organisation needed to change before developing action plans.

At St George's Healthcare NHS Trust, where I was Chief Executive at the time clinical governance was introduced, the questions that kept arising were, how do we decide what constitutes an acceptable standard of practice – and where do we go to find measurable standards? And how can we be sure that the standards we select will satisfy the extensive and growing array of organisations that will come and inspect us? The answer lies in the guidance produced by NICE. With our ability to engage with the NHS, professional bodies and patient advocate organisations, we can produce standards in which both clinicians and managers can have full confidence. They will know that we have developed them in a way that will meet the reasonable expectations of the scrutinisers.

The existence of a programme of authoritative national guidance is an essential element in the successful implementation of clinical governance. Without it, consistent standards will elude the NHS, and clinical governance will become a guessing game for patients. Such an arrangement could not be reconciled with the concept of a national healthcare system.

References

1   *The Economist.* July 31–August 6 1999: 22.
2   Medline search, 1993 to present.
3   NHS and Community Care Act 1990.
4   Brahams D. Judicial review of refusal to fund treatment. *Lancet* 1995; 345(8951): 717.
5   *National Institute for Clinical Excellence. Guidance on the Use of Taxanes for Ovarian Cancer.* May 2000
6   NHS Executive. *Faster Access to Modern Treatment.* 1999.
7   National Institute for Clinical Excellence. *Referral Practice – A Guide to Appropriate Referral from General to Specialist Services.* June 2000.

▶12

Revalidation, Poor Performance and Clinical Governance

David Hatch

Introduction

Although staff within managed systems are governed by their contracts, healthcare professionals are also accountable to their regulatory bodies. Patients and doctors have a common interest in effective medical professionalism.1 For doctors in the UK, the General Medical Council (GMC) has been the regulatory body since its establishment in 1858, setting the educational requirements for entry onto the Medical Registrar and the professional standards expected of doctors once they are on it. Many doctors are not in managed systems and they are therefore solely accountable to the GMC for their professional performance. Originally, doctors could only be removed from the Register on grounds of serious professional misconduct. However, the health procedures, established in 1980, and the performance procedures, introduced in 1997, allowed the GMC to put conditions on the registration of doctors with seriously impaired health or seriously deficient performance and in the most severe cases to suspend these doctors' registration indefinitely.

The GMC made the professional standards required of doctors on the register more explicit in 1995 by the publication of the booklet Good Medical Practice (revised in 1998),2 and has introduced a number of other important initiatives. In 1996, it increased its non-medical membership from 10% to 25%, and in 1997 made eligibility for consultant posts in the National Health Service dependent on entry onto the newly introduced Specialist Register. Further recommendations on postgraduate medical education were published in 19973 and 19984 as part of the GMC's ongoing review on standards of medical practice. Many of these initiatives have been developed in conjunction with the medical Royal Colleges, specialist associations, universities and postgraduate deans.

Members of the public understandably expect the Medical Register to indicate those doctors who are currently fit to practice, and many are surprised to learn that this has not been the case. Until recently, there has been no mechanism for assessing the conduct, health or performance of any doctor on the Medical Register unless allegations of serious deficiency against them are reported to the GMC. The Register's Principal List thus only provides a list of names of people who have at some time, possibly many decades ago, passed an accepted qualifying examination and satisfactorily completed a period of provisional or temporary registration and against whom nothing adverse is known by the GMC. Similarly, many doctors are on the Specialist Register by virtue of their consultant status, which may have been obtained many years ago. This is no longer adequate to satisfy public demand for assurances that doctors remain capable and safe throughout their practising lives.[5]

Despite the explicit professional obligation in *Good Medical Practice*[2] for doctors to act quickly to protect patients when a colleague may not be fit to practice, there is still a degree of reluctance among some doctors to 'blow the whistle' in this situation. It is clear, therefore, that any system that relies solely on the reporting of poor practice is unlikely to be sufficient in the long term to maintain public confidence in the profession. In addition, many doctors would welcome the opportunity to demonstrate that they are giving good medical care, and to be helped to correct any weaknesses promptly in a supportive environment.

In February 1999, the Council resolved that continued registration should be linked with regular active demonstration by all registered doctors that they remained fit to practice and up to date in their chosen field. There is, however, no evidence that periodic re-certification of credentials by some form of examination bears any relation to clinical performance, so the GMC has decided to adopt a performance-based system, which has become known as *revalidation*. The GMC is committed to having a worked-up model ready for approval by its Council in May 2001, and its consultation document was published in June 2000.[6] Such a system will have six core components:[5]

- A clear, ethical framework and, wherever possible, the use of explicit professional and clinical standards;

- Effective local professional regulation for maintaining good practice;

- Regular publication by the Royal Colleges and others of data showing doctors' involvement in continuing medical education (CME), audit, and other performance-related activities;

- Sound local arrangements for recognising dysfunctional doctors early and taking appropriate action;

- Well-defined criteria and pathways for referral to the GMC when severely dysfunctional doctors cannot or should not be managed locally;

- At all stages, practical help and support so that doctors who get into difficulties can be restored to full practice, wherever possible.

In a parallel development, the Government, in its June 1998 publication *A First Class Service – Quality in the New NHS*,[7] outlined its plans to introduce a system of clinical governance, a process by which each part of the NHS provides quality assurance for its clinical decisions. Backed by a new statutory duty of quality, it aims to introduce a system of continuous improvement into the operation of the whole NHS, encouraging life-long learning, strengthening professional self-regulation and identifying possible lapses in clinical quality at an early stage. Standards will be monitored by three new mechanisms: a Commission for Health Improvement (CHI), a National Framework for assessing performance and an annual national survey of patient and user experience of the NHS. Additionally, the Department of Health in England is consulting on ways of preventing, recognising and dealing with poor clinical performance of doctors working in the NHS through its publication *Supporting Doctors, Protecting Patients.*[8] The government has also taken steps to strengthen the independent healthcare sector.

Although these initiatives have not been developed as a 'knee jerk' response to recent high-profile examples of poor practice, the disproportionate media publicity that these cases have attracted has focused the minds of both politicians and doctors. It has demonstrated clearly the need to introduce strengthened and effective systems of regulation and quality assurance as quickly as possible. The introduction of an effective and simple system of revalidation, as outlined below, will be critical in ensuring that all doctors subject their practices to regular review and will be a touchstone of credibility for the GMC.

Revalidation and performance

Although at the time of writing the GMC's proposals on revalidation for all doctors are still subject to widespread consultation, their general shape is now becoming clear. The Council has decided that the evidence to demonstrate fitness to practice for doctors should be generated locally (Figure 12.1). The information required is likely

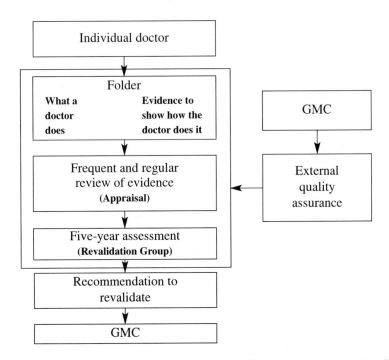

Fig. 12.1. The revalidation process. Reproduced with permission from the General Medical Council.

to include results of audit and other quality improvement methods, a record of continuing professional development (CPD), the views of a sample of patients, where appropriate, and views of colleagues. Local systems for generating and reviewing that evidence should be subject to periodic external peer review, and, wherever possible, existing and proposed systems should be used to keep the burden to a minimum. The GMC will, however, need to ensure that there are appropriate and effective revalidation arrangements for all registered doctors, irrespective of grade, specialty and employment status. Periodically, probably every five years, the doctor's folder will be assessed independently by a small revalidation group appointed by the GMC. It is suggested that this group would contain a minimum of three people, and might comprise two registered doctors (one of whom has personal knowledge of the doctor and one from the same field of practice) and a lay person independent of the organisation in which the doctor works. The revalidation decision must be objective, fair, transparent and free from discrimination.

On 1 October 1999, there were 193 366 doctors on the Register of whom 36 199 were on the Specialist Register. Registered doctors work in a wide variety of chosen fields, whilst some, for a variety of different reasons, do not practice at all and may opt to move to a register of unvalidated doctors. Some doctors are registered in more than one specialty and not all are members of Royal Colleges, faculties or specialist associations. The majority of doctors in active clinical practice in the UK work in some capacity within the NHS at various grades and in various specialities. The NHS can be split roughly into two main areas: hospital practice and general practice. The former category includes consultants, non-consultant career-grade doctors, clinical assistants and doctors-in-training. The latter category contains GP principals and non-principals, and GP registrars.

There are also doctors employed within the Department of Health, the NHS Executive, Health Authorities, Boards and Trusts who may not be engaged in the direct clinical care of patients. This group includes doctors employed in public health medicine and some medical directors. In addition to the NHS, there are a number of other public sector areas in which doctors work, such as the prison service and armed forces. There also are many doctors who work outside the NHS, for example those engaged in full-time private medical practice, occupational health doctors in private companies, doctors employed by the pharmaceutical and other industries, and ships' doctors. Some doctors undertake clinical work for more than one organisation at the same time or may work independently outside their main area of employment.

Locum doctors perform an extremely valuable function and work in most areas of medical practice. A recent audit commission report on locum doctors states that on a typical day, there are around 3500 doctors working as locums in England and Wales. Some doctors are only engaged in active medical practice on a part-time basis, and where they practice only intermittently it may be difficult for them to provide evidence of their fitness to practice. Others are not in active clinical practice but may require continued registration, such as those retained by firms of solicitors to provide medico-legal reports, those employed in medico-political work or holding high national office, such as the President of the GMC and the four Chief Medical Officers.

A separate issue is raised by those doctors who may be employed for a time in primary administrative capacities but who may wish to return to medical practice at a later date – for example, undergraduate or postgraduate deans. Of the 191 682 doctors on the Principal List in October 1999, 165 607 had registered addresses in the UK and 26 075 had registered addresses elsewhere. It does not necessarily follow that a registered address in the UK signifies that a doctor works in the UK or that an address abroad means a doctor lives and works abroad, but for those who choose to spend a significant period of their time overseas, suitable evidence of fitness to practice is likely to be incomplete. Some doctors choose, for a variety of reasons, to take a career break of variable duration after which they may wish to return to active clinical practice.

It is not clear how many doctors on the Register have retired from medical practice, and at present there is no record of date of birth on the Register. On the assumption that the majority of medical practitioners qualify at the age of 25, deducting 25 from the year of qualification suggests that approximately 30 000 registered doctors are over the age of 70. There is no information available to indicate how many of these doctors are involved in any form of clinical practice or exercising any of the privileges of registration. Anecdotal evidence suggests that retired doctors prescribe not infrequently for family and friends.

It is clear from the above analysis that the development of revalidation systems for all categories of doctors is not going to be an easy task. In addressing this problem, the GMC has decided that revalidation will be based on a demonstration of the attributes of a good doctor as set out in its guidance *Good Medical Practice*.[2] Whilst many of these attributes are generic, some Royal Colleges and specialist associations have published guidance on how the principles in the guidance apply in the particular practice circumstances of their members. Currently, these include the Royal Colleges of Anaesthetists,[9] General Practitioners,[10] Obstetricians and Gynaecologists,[11] Radiologists[12] and Ophthalmologists.[13] Others are in the process of developing such guidance, and all are being encouraged to do so. The Academy of Medical Royal Colleges also has produced a number of working papers on the key issues raised by revalidation.

There are three stages proposed for the revalidation process:

a) A folder of information describing what the doctor does and how well he/she does it. This will be reviewed regularly.
b) Periodic revalidation – a recommendation by an independent group of medical and lay people that the doctor remains fit to practise, or that his/her registration should be reviewed by the GMC.
c) Action by the GMC – in the majority of cases, revalidation of the doctor's entry in the Register; in a minority, detailed investigation under the GMC's fitness-to-practise procedures.

Existing and planned local fitness-to-practise arrangements

Revalidation should be based, as far as possible, on existing and proposed local quality arrangements. Some of these are outlined below.

a) Doctors in training

Revalidation arrangements for doctors in training should be based, as far as possible, on existing arrangements for their monitoring, appraisal and assessment. If these arrangements are working properly, the revalidation of a doctor in training who is making satisfactory process either at senior house officer, GP registrar or specialist registrar grade should be straightforward. For the process to be acceptable, however, it must be seen to be underpinned by *Good Medical Practice*[2] more explicitly than it sometimes is and the introduction of a lay element into the assessment will need to be considered. The GMC has set out in its publication *The New Doctor*[3] both the required content of PHRO (pre-registration house officer) training and the composition of formal educational programmes. In its publication *The Early Years*,[4] it has given guidance on the generic knowledge, understanding and skills that must be covered during the senior house officer period of training. Specialist registrars, whose training is becoming increasingly competency based, are required to complete a record of in-training assessment (RITA). This provides a record of the annual review and of the doctor's progress through the training programme and the grade. It is normally completed by the trainee and the postgraduate dean each year. General practice training is delivered within practices by GP trainers accredited by the Joint Committee on Postgraduate Training for General Practice, which sets the standards for all GP training. However, locum, assistant and deputising GPs who are eligible to practise by virtue of their acquired rights may have had no training whatsoever in general practise. GP registrars in the UK commencing their training on or after 30 January 1998 must have passed a test of competence, known as summative assessment, before they can work unsupervised.

b) Career-grade doctors

Career-grade doctors are encouraged to participate in CME and CPD initiatives, many of which are coordinated by the Royal Colleges and faculties. Doctors who are trainers also may obtain some measure of feedback on their performance. All NHS doctors are required to participate in clinical audit, and involvement in national clinical audits and confidential enquiries will become an essential component of clinical governance. There have been almost no attempts, however, to require doctors to relate their ongoing education to their own areas of practice, or to attempt to identify and remedy areas of weakness. Many CME and CPD programmes are voluntary, so that those who most need them may well decide not to participate.

bi) NHS hospital doctors

Regular review of performance is likely to be an essential requirement for all doctors taking part in the revalidation process. Appraisal has become accepted for trainees in the NHS and has been adopted by universities for many years. It is now generally accepted that annual appraisal will become part of all NHS career-grade contracts, and discussions are taking place between the NHS Executive and the GMC to ensure that this will be acceptable for revalidation. Doctors working outside the NHS will need to take part in similar processes. Although the purpose of appraisal is formative, it will provide an important opportunity to support revalidation by a review of the doctor's folder, ensuring that the information in it is accurate and sufficient, identifying gaps and difficulties to be addressed, and highlighting any contribution made by environmental factors towards the doctor's performance. Appraisal will provide an opportunity to facilitate or arrange any developmental or remedial action required and agree a personal development plan for the coming year.

In exceptional circumstances, doctors undertaking appraisals will have to take appropriate steps to protect patients from dangerously poor performance, under their professional duties to the GMC. However, in the vast majority of cases regular annual appraisal will allow a doctor to accumulate the evidence required within the five-year time frame for revalidation and ensure that there are no surprises at the end of this period. Some Royal Colleges and specialist associations are already providing guidance on the nature of the information required for their members in the revalidation folder; helping to define recommended standards for audit and offering help when problems arise. The Joint Committee on Good Practice of the Royal College and the Association of Anaesthetists has devised a list of recommended core topics to help anaesthetists target their CME and CPD. Some Royal Colleges have produced audit 'recipe books' to help their members target their audit activities.[14,15]

bii) General practitioners

Most GPs are independent contractors. In common with their hospital colleagues, however, they are subject to central guidance from the Department of Health on a variety of practice and procedural issues. The Joint Committee on Postgraduate Training in General Practice (JCPTGP) has set out the standards it expects individual GP trainers to meet, and identifies the expected attributes of a training practice. Recognition as a GP trainer is time-limited, and trainers are expected to be willing to have their clinical abilities assessed by their peers. Participation in CME programmes is part of this process and trainers are required to demonstrate ways in which they organise their CME. Some deaneries are encouraging trainers to have a personal learning plan, which can be reviewed on inspection visits.

The Royal College of General Practitioners has attempted to define some of the attributes of an excellent and an unacceptable GP, has set up a working group on revalidation and operates a number of different CPD arrangements. It plans to introduce a system of time-limited accredited professional development (APD) which is separate from revalidation but will be closely related. It will cover four main areas: keeping up to date; ability to communicate; improving care; and professional behaviour. This will be a voluntary system for GPs, allowing them to demonstrate explicitly their commitment to life-long learning that will be based on the principle of peer review and measured quality improvement. Success in membership and fellowship of the Royal College by Assessment of Performance would, however, provide substantial evidence for both APD and revalidation.

biii) Doctors in the private and independent healthcare sector

The Private Practice Forum has set out the standards that it expects of all doctors working in private practice.[16] These standards were devised under the auspices of the Academy of Medical Royal Colleges, the British Medical Association, the

Independent Healthcare Association and the Association of British Insurers. All private doctors are expected to maintain the current knowledge and skills relevant to their area of speciality and to undertake CME in accordance with the standards set down by the appropriate Royal College or faculty. All private doctors also are expected to ensure that they participate in CPD and produce three-year reviews of professional development plans. The management boards of the private hospitals are becoming increasingly careful in checking the professional standards of those doctors to whom they grant admitting rights to their hospitals. Most doctors working in the private sector are also employed in the NHS and will therefore be subject to the appraisal systems for hospital doctors described above. Every private doctor is expected to participate actively in clinical audits, and medical advisory committees should ensure that mandatory audit is carried out, reviewing the results and advising management on any action needed within their hospitals.

biv) Doctors in the armed forces
The Ministry of Defence has made an arrangement with the Department of Health for the work of the CHI to be extended to the armed forces. It is also reviewing its practices to ensure that they take account of clinical governance initiatives through liaison with the Department of Health, NHS Executive and GMC. Consultants serving in the armed forces are, like their NHS colleagues, expected to participate in CPD and CME, to develop their skills and keep up to date, and to participate in clinical audit. The JCPTGP is responsible for the approval of all armed services GP training posts and inspects the armed services as part of its accreditation visiting process.

All doctors working in the armed forces are subject to an annual appraisal process on the same lines as their non-medical peers. This is undertaken by their line manager, with supplementary medical input where necessary.

bv) Doctors in the prison services
In a recent NHS Executive and HM Prison Service report,[17] a future strategy for CPD is recommended. It proposes that plans will be in line with present recommendations from the NHS and the Royal Colleges. In the future, prison doctors will adopt the quality systems set out in the NHS document *A First Class Service. Quality in the NHS*,[7] including appraisal and audit.

c) Locum doctors
The NHS Executive has issued a code of practice on the appointment and employment of locum doctors in an attempt to improve quality control of this group of practitioners. It recommends that a full report on locum doctors should be prepared at the end of each locum period, identifying training needs as well as knowledge, attitudes, relationships and personal qualities of the individual. These reports are likely to form the basis for the locum doctor's revalidation folder, although more work needs to be done to identify mechanisms to enable locum doctors to take part in audit and CPD and to receive the benefits of regular annual appraisal. This group of doctors may well provide the greatest challenge for revalidation.

d) Doctors working outside managed systems

Whilst the principles of revalidation will be the same for all doctors, there will be a greater onus on those working exclusively outside managed systems to make their own arrangements. They will not have the benefit of arrangements that result from contractual agreements. They will still be expected to keep a folder of information and identify a doctor who is prepared to review it on a regular basis in between the revalidation decisions. They may be able to receive help from the relevant Medical Royal College.

Existing and planned external peer review processes

Healthcare services in the UK are subject to a variety of external review systems which, if working properly, should feed in to the revalidation process. These include The Clinical Standards Advisory Group, the CHI, The Clinical Standards Board For Scotland, The Clinical Negligence Scheme for Trusts, The Welsh Risk Pool, The Mental Health Act Commission (Mental Welfare Commission in Scotland), surveys conducted by community health councils and other health councils and regulatory processes carried out within the independent healthcare sector. Healthcare organisations also have increasingly used a variety of accreditation bodies to assess their level of performance in relation to established standards and to help implement ways of continuously improving the healthcare system. The UK Accreditation Forum, formed in 1998, has identified organisations that are devoted to improving the quality of healthcare by providing standards based on assessment of specialty services or organisations. Many accreditation services focus on process and systems and not on performance of individuals; it is well recognised that good doctors can be struggling within dysfunctional teams and *vice versa*. There is no reason, however, why the contribution of individuals to the overall performance of organisations should not be recognised in their revalidation folder. Similarly, organisations wishing to be accredited under, for example, the Accreditation and Development of Health Records Programme are likely to take steps to ensure that individuals within the organisation subscribe to the required standards of record-keeping.

Some specialist societies have developed peer review schemes and others are considering doing so. That organised by the British Thoracic Society was one of the first of such schemes and has been running since 1992. This scheme is currently being revised and upgraded and may become mandatory if the Royal College concludes that the review should become part of the clinical governance process and if the scheme is adequately funded. Such schemes may be more relevant to the development of local profiling processes than to the external review of them, however.

The GMC has drafted assessment criteria for the external peer review of local profiling systems. Where appraisal systems exist, it should be relatively straightforward to assure their suitability for revalidation; for example, in the NHS in England and Wales it should be possible for the CHI to assure their quality. The GMC proposes to identify a number of organisations that could help provide external quality assurance. Audit of the quality of processes will not be sufficient, however. It also will be necessary to check that the quality of recommendations made to the GMC is consistent with the evidence. One proposal is that within institutions that have satisfactory appraisal systems for reviewing performance, 1% of revalidation recommendations should be sampled on a five-year cycle. Where no routine appraisal exists, for example in the case of doctors working outside managed organisations, a larger sample of revalidation recommendations (possibly as high as 10%) should be audited.

At the time of writing, a number of questions about the revalidation process remain unanswered and these will not be resolved until the end of the consultation period. Questions arise about the extent and types of information that might be included in the revalidation folder, and whether, for example, complaints against a doctor, together with their outcome, should be included. Opinions are being sought about both the medical and lay membership of the Revalidation Group responsible for making the final recommendation to the GMC and the systems for the revalidation of locum doctors, retired doctors, doctors working abroad and those taking a career break need further development. The GMC is also inviting views about which, if any, of the privileges of registration it would be safe to allow unrevalidated doctors to retain.

Managing poor performance

Handling poor performance locally

The GMC's publication *Maintaining Good Medical Practice*[18] describes the principles under which doctors should be referred to the GMC. These will continue to apply at all times – not just when the doctor is due for a revalidation decision.

It has been agreed that doctors will not have their registration affected adversely by the revalidation process without going through one of the GMC's existing fitness-to-practise processes (conduct, health or performance), although doctors who fail to participate will be liable, after due process, to erasure. The decision by the local revalidation group will be a straightforward one of either to recommend revalidation or not. If there are concerns about a doctor that are not serious enough to affect the revalidation recommendation, the revalidation group will have a responsibility to point this out so that they can be addressed locally without delay. Doctors who are not recommended for revalidation will have the evidence for that decision assessed by GMC screeners who will decide whether or not the evidence justifies referral to one of the fitness-to-practise committees, where they will go through the same process as doctors who have been accused of serious deficiencies. They will have the same opportunities to defend themselves and the same rights of appeal as all doctors. If the evidence does not justify referral, the doctor's registration will be revalidated.

Since revalidation is a rolling process, with the revalidation decision probably being taken at five-yearly intervals, there should be plenty of opportunity for annual appraisal systems to identify gaps in the revalidation folders of individual doctors and for any action required to fill these gaps to be taken. Therefore, there should be no surprises at the end of the five-year period, as that small group of doctors who will not be recommended for revalidation are likely to have been identified well before this decision is made. Some doctors already will have been referred to the GMC under its fitness-to-practise arrangements, since if at any stage serious concerns are raised they should be addressed immediately.

In order to help ensure that local medical regulation based on the GMC's documents *Good Medical Practice*[2] and *Maintaining Good Medical Practice*[18] can be satisfactorily implemented, the GMC set up a working group under the chairmanship of Professor Siân Griffiths. This working group has developed a framework to enable those with local responsibilities to assess whether the professional requirements in *Good Medical Practice*[2] and *Maintaining Good Medical Practice*,[18] which apply to all doctors, are monitored at every stage of the medical career and to identify areas where this is not occurring. The framework is not prescriptive but allows different organisations to adjust it according to their own priorities and particular concerns. It is not designed to assess how individual doctors are practising but to enable an assessment of local systems to ensure the application of the principles set out by the GMC. The framework can be applied at all stages of a doctor's career pathway – from selection into medical training as an undergraduate to reattainment of career-grade status. The report of the working group identifies four possible activities at each stage of the career pathway where the framework could be applied. These are appointment, development, departure and remediation. The application of this framework provides one way of ensuring that whenever the performance of a doctor is assessed it is against the GMC's template of *Good Medical Practice* (Figure 12.2). The adoption of such a template by managers within the NHS and private sector, GP principals and partners responsible for employing locums and assistants, university medical schools, deaneries, the medical Royal Colleges, Specialist Training Authority and Joint Committee for Postgraduate Training of General Practitioners would provide a tangible link between clinical governance and revalidation to ensure the continuing development and assessment of professional standards of all doctors throughout their careers.

Links between revalidation and clinical governance

For quality assurance and improvement to be robust and effective, these professionally led and contractually driven initiatives must fit together like pieces of a jigsaw. In the words of the Chief Medical Officer, Professor Liam Donaldson, 'We are not playing one club golf.' Each initiative has complementary advantages and disadvantages. Clinical governance can take swift action, proportional to the size of the problem, but cannot easily determine appropriate professional standards, deal with the private sector or prevent dangerous doctors from practising elsewhere. Revalidation, on the other hand, can provide a clear set of professional standards to support good practice, and remove dangerous doctors from all forms of practise requiring registration, but cannot currently take very rapid action or deliver remedial solutions. Despite inevitable tensions between the profession and the Executive, there does seem to be a willingness to ensure that this close interlinkage takes place. At the time of writing, there are early signs of a change in balance in relation to the professional regulation of doctors. Employers, whether in the state or private sector, are increasingly taking

	Good clinical care	Maintaining good medical practice	Teaching and training	Maintaining trust	Working with colleagues	Probity	Health
Appointment							
Appraisal							
Departure							
Remedial action							

Fig. 12.2. Attributes. (The seven categories of attributes cover all fourteen duties of a doctor outlined in *Good Medical Practice*.[2]) Reproduced with permission from the General Medical Council.

responsibility under their new statutory duty of quality for the early detection and management of poor performance. A system of appraisal will be a cornerstone of this new development and will hopefully be based on the profession's own template of 'good medical practice' required for continuing registration. At the same time, efforts are being made to change the culture in which doctors work at a local level. The 'Three Wise Men' scheme has been shown to have serious weaknesses[19] and needs to be replaced. Some Trusts are experimenting with alternative informal schemes to help deal at an early stage with conduct, health or performance issues. Offers of sabbatical leave may encourage doctors to reflect on their performance and develop their knowledge and skills. An environment is needed which promotes quality improvement, recognises the inevitability of even good doctors making errors and encourages openness and honesty about the performance of individuals and clinical teams. Such an environment, in which weaknesses can be identified and individuals can be helped to improve rather than be blamed, may offer the best chance for sustained quality improvement in healthcare.

References

1   Irvine D. The performance of doctors. I: Professionalism and self regulation in a changing world. *BMJ* 1997; 314: 1540–1542.
2   General Medical Council. *Good Medical Practice.* London, 1998.
3   General Medical Council. *The New Doctor: Recommendations on General Clinical Training.* London, 1997.
4   General Medical Council. *The Early Years.* London, 1998.
5   Irvine D. The performance of doctors. II: Maintaining good practice, protecting patients from poor performance. *BMJ* 1997; 314: 1613–1615.
6   General Medical Council. *Revalidating Doctors: Ensuring Standards, Securing the Future.* London, 2000.
7   Department of Health. *A First Class Service. Quality in the NHS.* London: The Stationery Office, 1998.
8   Department of Health. *Supporting Doctors, Protecting Patients.* London: The Stationery Office, 1999.
9   Royal College of Anaesthetists and Association of Anaesthetists of Great Britain and Ireland. Good Practice. A Guide for Departments of Anaesthesia. London, 1998.
10 Royal College of General Practitioners and BMA GP Committee. *Good Medical Practice for General Practitioners.* London, 1999.
11 Royal College of Obstetricians and Gynaecologists. *Maintaining Good Medical Practice in Obstetrics and Gynaecology.* London, 1999.
12 Board of the Faculty of Clinical Radiologists. The Royal College of Radiologists. *Good Practice Guide for Clinical Radiologists.* London, 1999.
13 The Royal College of Ophthalmology. *Quality Development Programme. Guidance for Clinical Governance in Ophthalmology.* London, 1999.
14 The Royal College of Anaesthetists. Lack JA, White L, Thoms, G, Rollin A-M. *Raising the Standard: A Compendium of Audit Recipes for Continuous Improvement in Anaesthesia.* London, 1999.
15 Godwin R, deLacey G, Manhire A. *Clinical Audit in Radiology: 100+ Recipes.* London: The Royal College of Radiologists, 1996.
16 Private Practice Forum. *A Guide to Standards in Private Practice.* 1997.
17 HM Prison Service and NHS Executive *The Future Organisation of Prison Healthcare.* London, 1999.
18 General Medical Council. *Maintaining Good Medical Practice.* London, 1998.
19 Rosenthal MM. *The Incompetent Doctor: Behind Closed Doors.* Buckingham: Open University Press, 1995.

►13

Control Assurance

Tim Scott

Management systems, governance and controls assurance

The establishment of the management systems of an NHS Trust follows a simple, well-understood path. After the Secretary of State appoints the Chair, he/she and the other nonexecutives appoint a Chief Executive and the rest of the Trust board.

The executive team then will draw up a system of delegation, including, but not limited to, a structure of accountability, and propose the adoption of this. The formalisation of these arrangements, including the agreement of roles and responsibilities and of job descriptions, means that the Trust board agrees to a specific scheme. A key element of these arrangements will usually be the delegation of financial powers, traditionally set out in the Trust's standing orders (SOs) and standing financial instructions (SFIs).

All Trusts adopt a substructure – sometimes around clinical clusters, with clinical directors, sometimes on geographic lines with unit or patch managers. In any event, a clear line of accountability exists between managers and the chief executive officer (CEO).

The crucial question for Trust boards thereafter is not, 'Who is accountable?', but 'How are they accountable?' That is, what reporting arrangements are in place and how can the board be assured that the management arrangements work and are effective? The key to this is to look at parallels between the well-established world of financial governance and the newly emerging world of clinical governance.

Inevitably, there is considerable focus, particularly from the press, the legal system and the public, on the issue of minimum standards. Wherever our duties of care fall below these standards, we can – and should – expect public concern. NHS fraud in both secondary and primary care sectors continues to be an issue, as does clinical negligence. Much that goes wrong at this level can be described as system failure, rather than people failure but nevertheless the popular press' image is always of the 'rogue' practitioner. One important aspect of beginning to see clinical governance and controls assurance as holistic is to understand that rogue behaviour is likely to occur across the spectrum. That is, an individual who is negligent in a clinical way also may fail to observe scrupulous standards of financial probity. It is worth remembering that Al Capone was only ever convicted for tax evasion.

The development of controls assurance

Colin Reeves was NHS Executive Director of Finance from 1994 to date (ie 2001). He worked for two different political administrations and provided a level of continuity during times of rapid change in the NHS. His solid and lasting achievements during this period can be seen as twofold:

▶ a considerably healthier finance function, with high levels of recruitment, morale and qualified staff, and

▶ firm establishment of controls assurance, which has made the NHS not just a leader in the public sector but probably one of the world leaders for large complex organisations.

He describes the approach that the Department took as comprising three simple steps:

▶ Introduction of the accounting officer concept.

▶ Strengthening of the internal audit function.

▶ Establishment of controls assurance.

In 1994, the understanding of accountability for central government departments was that the permanent secretary was the 'accounting officer', accountable for all expenditure to Parliament and in particular to the Public Accounts Committee. The Department of Health and NHS Executive devolved those responsibilities to chief executives and introduced the notion of 'dual accountability', so that the chief executive of Trusts are now accountable to their Chair and the Trust board, and also to Parliament and the Public Accounts Committee, for the financial affairs of the organisation. This formal devolution of accountability not only clarified the arrangements within the NHS but also gave chief executives a keen interest in developing the necessary mechanisms to give themselves and their board some assurance in this area.

The key to strengthening the internal systems lay in the internal audit function of the finance department. Typically for a Trust, this would consist of between four and six dedicated staff working to the director of finance. The problem was that for many years, this had been a 'low status' job within finance itself, the general percentage of qualified staff was low and there was little benchmarking or peer review. Over the years, we have seen the development of consortia providing internal audit functions to a number of Trusts, resulting in much larger internal audit departments. These can now range anywhere from 10–50 people and not only provide economy of scale and holiday cover but also – and more importantly – support an increasing degree of professionalism, peer review and pride. Thus, the human resources component so critical to improving assurance systems has been enhanced thoughtfully and systematically.

The final step was to begin to introduce specific controls assurance standards into the accounts. In 1988/1989, the first five required standards were introduced. The department set out areas that must be covered in the annual financial report, where Trusts would have to demonstrate that robust systems were in place and offer these systems for scrutiny by external audit. The record demonstrates how well the NHS achieved this – over the past five years, only one set of Trust accounts have been qualified by external auditors on one occasion.

The strategy was to build gradually from a firm base in controls to other areas of organisational management systems. The triangle, reproduced as Figure 13.1, formed a standard part of the departmental slide set during this era. Lovingly known as 'the wigwam', it tries to illustrate the relationship between the basic financial controls, the nonclinical and nonfinancial areas and those of clinical systems. Although custom and practice have resulted in a fairly clear understanding of systems which are financial as opposed to other areas (although value for money and some other areas might be debated), there is much less clarity regarding the rest of the triangle. As an example, systems of infectious disease control, although clearly clinical in nature, have been included in 'nonfinancial' and 'nonclinical'. Since the whole purpose of an NHS Trust is to provide clinical services, however, all systems aim in some capacity to this overarching goal; and clearly, therefore, this is a division of convenience, rather than an absolute one.

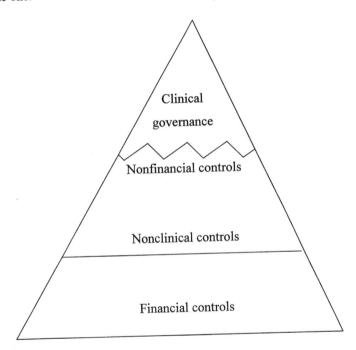

Fig. 13.1. 'The wigwam'

By 2000, the annual accounts covered organisational control standards in nonfinancial, nonclinical areas, including, for example, fire safety and medical equipment. The 16 standards set out by the department all had a set of underpinning criteria. Again taking fire safety as an example, these included establishment of a documented Trust policy, the nomination of a Trust board executive director with specific responsibility for fire safety and the undertaking of a fire drill at least once a year. Indeed, formal standards were introduced for each specific area that the NHS was required to systematically respond to.

What are the drives for seeing explicit links with clinical governance? From a financial perspective, the rapidly growing figure of outstanding negligence claims, currently standing at £3.2billion, must be acknowledged as a major concern. This single factor, and the increasing level of public concern about the monitoring of clinical standards, are the key drivers.

Nevertheless, the basis of the approach to governance adopted worldwide and promoted within the NHS has been of self-assessment and verification. In the end, Trusts themselves need to tackle these areas pro-actively, and the Department needs to provide every form of support that it can to that self-assessment. Of course, the department, Secretary of State and the wider public do require some form of independent verification also. The complexity of the current situation is demonstrated in Figure 13.2. We can see the wide variety of independent and external bodies with roles to play in the verification of assurance. There is as yet, however, no clear and shared understanding of how this overlap is to be tackled.

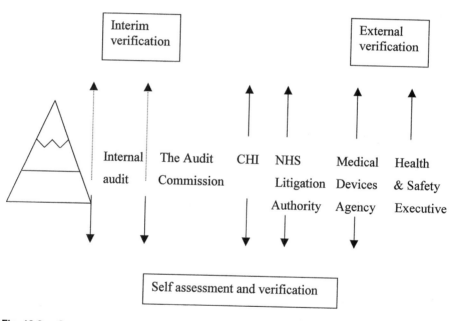

Fig. 13.2. Governance assessment

To describe controls assurance in the NHS as an industry would be to belittle the efforts of the finance function. There is a very considerable and solid body of work undertaken and documented on controls assurance in the NHS, much of which is readily available through the dedicated website (URL http://www.doh.gov.uk/riskman.htm). An indication of the depth and substance of this work is that the issue of guidelines has now moved from printed paper to CD-ROM. This chapter is not intended to provide a complete overview and insight into that work. Rather, it attempts to give some of the history and background to controls assurance, to consider the (inevitable) convergence with clinical governance, to look at practical local first steps for NHS Trusts and primary care organisations (PCOs) to take in supporting this convergence. It also suggests that an increased focus on clinical teams and systems to support review and assure the working of teams is inherent in a holistic vision of governance.

The intellectual underpinning to controls assurance within the NHS should not be underestimated. The NHS arguably has one of the most sophisticated approaches worldwide to controls assurance. Following the Cadbury Report[1] and subsequent developments within the commercial sector, the NHS has drawn thoughtfully on the best that is available worldwide. American research, Australian standards and Canadian guidance all have been reviewed, and a widespread approach of expert committees, practitioner networks, websites, newsletters and other devices has ensured that there has been a positive and ongoing dialogue between theory and practice.

Parallels between financial and clinical management systems, governance and assurance

This section sets out a number of parallels between financial governance and clinical governance. It suggests that lessons and skills may be transferable from the well-established area of financial management and financial governance and that not only skill transfers but also shared working may be a useful support for Trusts.

The definition of clinical governance, first set out in the White Paper *A First Class Service*,[2] and subsequently re-iterated in the *BMJ*,[3] is as follows:

What is clinical governance?

Clinical Governance can be defined as a framework* through which NHS organisations are accountable for continuously improving the quality of their services and safeguarding high standards of care by creating an environment in which excellence in clinical care will flourish.

A First Class Service, page 33

It sets out quite clearly that what is involved is a way in which NHS organisations, particularly Trusts and increasingly, one imagines, primary care groups/trusts (PCGs/PCTs), are accountable. (It is important to note that this refers to the accountability of *organisations*, not the individual people within them.) For what are these organisations accountable, then? Two things:

▶ A bottom line: 'There are standards and we can put our hands on our hearts and say that no-one falls below those standards'; and

▶ A continuing search for improvement: 'We constantly strive in a systematic way to improve performance'.

---

* The word 'framework' from the original White Paper was replaced by 'system' in the *BMJ* article.[3]

Those from a finance background may already hear resonances with the core duties of the finance function. The bottom line for finance is probity – the NHS is funded by public money and we must be able to account for every penny that is spent in a transparent and open way and be able to assure people that no corruption or embezzlement has taken place. However, any director of finance who ran their Trust on this basis would quickly come to grief. They might be able to account for every penny but unless they also sought value for money they would almost certainly overspend. The other component of the function of finance is constantly to chase the chimera of value for money, but this is like trying to reach the end of the rainbow. You never can be absolutely sure that you achieve optimal value – all you can hope for is to have achieved best value in a particular context at a particular time.

How, then, do the director of finance and the finance staff set about this task? The simple answer is that they don't. They put in place a collection of systems and support to enable management to achieve these objectives. Anyone who has ever held a budget will be aware of SOs and SFIs, part of the finance 'bible' which spells out in each Trust what the rules are (eg what level of purchase is allowable by any one officer, at what point the Trust needs to go out to tender for things, and so on).

Finance helps the organisation to achieve the objectives of probity and value for money by devising and reviewing such financial systems.

In presenting this parallel to medical directors of Trusts, I have often been greeted with hollow laughter at this point. 'Give me the resources of the director of finance and I'll run the clinical governance system for you,' they say. Let's look at the typical finance department and begin to analyse who is undertaking these governance tasks. If we discount those staff involved in paying bills, wages and salaries, we are left with two groups of staff:

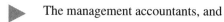 The management accountants, and

The internal audit staff.

Management accountants work to support the managers of the organisation, typically clinical directors and their business managers, in taking forward their plans and reviewing reality against plan (or actual against budget in financial terms). The financial internal audit staff review the financial systems on behalf of the Trust. For example, throughout a Trust there will be a variety of petty cash tins and a system of filling in slips, chits and having the float re-imbursed on a regular basis, which needs checking. However, it is unlikely that you can steal very much money from petty cash, and so this system will be checked on a relatively infrequent basis. On the other hand, it is quite possible to steal very large amounts of money from the payroll system, and systems of this high level of risk will need auditing far more frequently and more thoroughly. Nevertheless, all systems at some point need to be reviewed.

What is the process of system review? Clearly, the starting point must be adequate documentation of existing systems. In the 1960s, these were done on large rolls of paper as flow charts; nowadays, more sophisticated computer tools provide the same approach. Internal audit staff then will review what really happens against the formal specified system, checking for compliance (do people actually do what the system expects that they will do?) and effectiveness (even if people do comply, does that achieve the desired effect?)

In structural terms, all Trusts have a finance subcommittee of the Trust board usually chaired by a nonexecutive member of the Trust board, and the internal audit plan, which would include 20% contingency for unforeseeable problems, and would be reviewed and subsequently adopted by such a body.

So, we have a plan that has been approved by the organisation itself and particularly by the lay members of the organisation. This plan sets out how, over a period of time, a fixed resource will review all financial systems on a risk-weighted and comprehensive basis, including an allowance for unforeseeable events. How does this compare with the reviews of clinical governance systems? Is there a comprehensive clinical audit plan for the Trust? Is it properly risk-weighted but will nevertheless review all clinical areas over a period of time? Do only a minority of Trusts have anything as systematic as that suggested here?

In continuing to draw this parallel, whilst recognising the very different nature of clinical quality and financial value for money, we nevertheless see a lead individual, the medical director or nursing director, inevitably working closely with their colleague, taking an overall responsibility within the Trust, just as the director of finance does, for devising and setting in place the management systems and monitoring these systems to ensure governance. These systems are delivered by management and in particular clinical directors and business managers, but monitored by internal resources to check for effectiveness and compliance.

Convergence

As the preceding sections have demonstrated, there is an inevitable convergence between the two relatively distinct initiatives known as clinical governance and controls assurance. What any NHS organisation needs is a coherent set of systems which, interlocking together, provide the board – and through the board the NHS Executive, Secretary of State and the wider public – with assurance that not only are clinical standards secured and the organisation has certain minimum baselines, but that also systems for continually seeking improvement (either in value for money or in clinical outcome) are in place and are systematically monitored.

At one end of the spectrum of systems, illustrated in Figure 13.3, we see the need to set absolute minimum standards. In finance terms, these are referred to as probity (ie that all spending can be accounted for and is authorised properly). In clinical terms, these denote minimum clinical standards and guarantees that all care is at minimum delivered according to these baseline standards. At the other end of the spectrum we see systematic approaches that are capable of being monitored to constantly strive to 'do the best we can with the resources we've got' (in other words, to constantly strive for value for money and for maximum clinical effectiveness and efficiency).

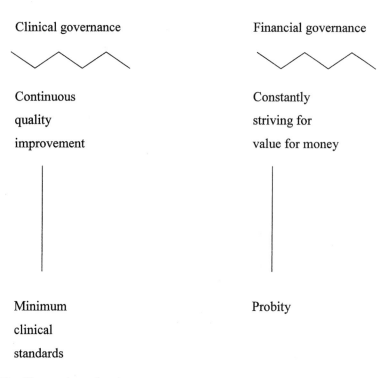

Fig. 13.3. The spectrum of systems

Practical steps support staff

As clinical governance has developed, particularly in acute Trusts, it has become clear that the medical director and director of nursing need to work together closely to ensure that governance systems are implemented and monitored appropriately. There are instances where they have pooled their resource – for example, those staff involved in clinical audit, those staff involved in quality control and others – to create a group of specialists who can design, implement and support managers in administering systems of local governance. As suggested earlier, there are major similarities between this work and the work that has been carried out by the internal audit department of finance specialists for many years. At an internal and technical level, therefore, each organisation might wish to begin to think about a group of specialists who have abilities to design, document and audit management systems, whether they are financial, nonfinancial/nonclinical or clinical. One model for the reporting and accountability arrangements for such a group is set out in Figure 13.4. Many directors of finance would be horrified to think of the financial internal audit staff not working to their direction. Nevertheless, the degree of independence needed by internal audit has always been recognised, as has been the capability of the head of internal audits to access either a chief executive or Chair, if, in their view, it is deemed necessary and appropriate.

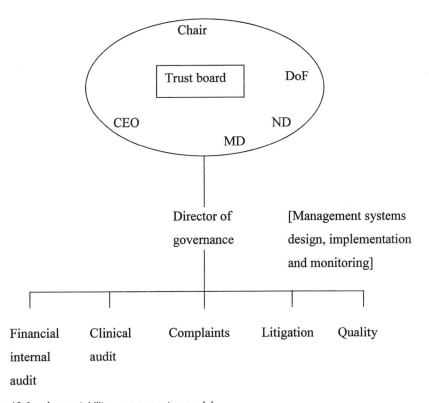

Fig. 13.4. Accountability arrangement: a model

Cultural issues

There are distinct cultural issues to be considered explicitly and tackled in the overlap and convergence of controls assurance and clinical governance. Finance is at heart a control discipline. On the other hand, clinical governance has been, slowly and cautiously, accepted by clinical staff, particular doctors, on the basis that it does address questions about striving for excellence and is not purely and simply a disciplinary or control system. In other words, clinical governance systems need to demonstrate often their contribution to continual improvement in order for the control system elements to be acceptable.

Summary

There is an inevitable convergence between controls assurance and clinical governance, and executive members of Trust boards will need to develop a holistic view of governance arrangements for the organisation as a whole. The design implementation and support of those systems, as well as their regular review, is currently likely to be undertaken by various groups within the organisation. Trusts should consider formulating a strategy for carefully and thoughtfully bringing these governance systems support groups together and taking a corporate view of the development of governance systems within the organisation.

Even without the influence of controls assurance, clinical governance will, of necessity, develop from its current relatively amateur and loosely documented arrangements into a much more substantial body of guidance and systems. Trusts will need to work hard to preserve the spirit of clinical governance and the constant striving for clinical improvements whilst delivering the more formal elements associated with minimum standards.

References

1   Sir Adrian Cadbury (Chair). Report of the Committee on the Financial Aspects of Corporate Governance, December 1992. See URL: http://www.ecgn.ulb.ac.be/ ecgn/docs/codes/cadbury.pdf.
2   Liam Donaldson. *A First Class Service. Quality in the New NHS.* London: HMSO, 1998. See URL: http://www.doh.gov.uk/newnhs/quality.htm.
3   Scally G, Donaldson LJ. Clinical governance and the drive for quality improvement in the new NHS in England. *BMJ* 1998; 317: 61–65.

►14

Guide to Sources

*Rosemary Hittinger, Dorothy Gregson, Jane Cartwright, Julie Glanville
and Sue Johnson*

Clinical Audit

> The systematic and critical analysis of the quality of clinical care, including the
> procedures used for diagnosis, treatment and care, the associated use of resources
> and the resulting outcomes and quality of life for the patient.
>
> **Working For Patients, 1989**

> Clinical audit is a multi-disciplinary activity which uses peer evaluation to
> demonstrate and improve the quality of patient care.

Organisations:

Association for Quality in Healthcare

Clinical Audit is only one of the special interest/focus groups provided by this
organisation, which was established to bring together individuals and organisations
who have an interest in continuously improving the quality of healthcare in the UK
and in furthering the knowledge related to the subject of quality in healthcare. It was
established to promote measurable and continuous improvement in the quality of
healthcare for the benefit of the public; also working to provide professional
recognition of healthcare workers with specific responsibility for quality matters.

It provides:

► A regular journal (*Healthcare Quality*)

► Regular branch/special interest meetings

► An educational programme.

Association for Quality in Healthcare

Portland House   **Tel:** 0118 981 6666
Aldermaston Park   **Fax:** 0118 981 9801
Reading   **URL:** www.aqh-uk.com
Berks RG7 4HR

Clinical Audit Association

This was the first professional audit organisation – established 1991 – to provide
support for healthcare professionals working in this field and to provide a focus for the
development and promotion of clinical audit in the UK. It was responsible for

pioneering work on systematic identification of occupational standards for healthcare professionals working in this field.

It provides:

▶ Regular newsletter *Network*

▶ A flexible learning programme leading to a National Certificate in Clinical Audit.

Clinical Audit Association Ltd.

Cleethorpes Business Centre **Tel/fax:** 01472 210 682
Jackson Place **e-mail:** pmkent@the-caa-ltd.demon.co.uk;
Wilton Road **URL:** http://www.the-caa-ltd.demon.co.uk
Humberston,
North East Lincolnshire DN36 4AS

Clinical Resource and Audit Group (CRAG)

This is the lead body within the Scottish Executive Health Department, promoting clinical effectiveness in Scotland. CRAG's remit touches on a wide range of issues concerned with the quality of clinical care, including clinical audit and national audit projects.

CRAG
Scottish Executive Health Department **Tel:** 0131 244 3471
St Andrew's House **Fax:** 0131 244 2989
Edinburgh EH1 3DG **URL:** www.show.scot.nhs.uk/crag

National Institute of Clinical Excellence (NICE)

This was set up as a Special Health Authority on 1 April 1999 to promote clinical- and cost-effectiveness through robust and reliable guidance on current best practice.
NICE
90 Long Acre **Tel:** 020 7849 3444; fax: 020 7849 3127
London WC2E 9RZ **e-mail:** nice@nice.nhs.uk; URL: www.nice.org.uk/nice-web
This useful website has lists of Sentinel Clinical Audit Projects and links to Royal Colleges and bodies receiving core Clinical Audit Funding as well as a description of the current work programme.

Audit (and associated) activities of the Royal Colleges and Professional Associations:

Not all of the Royal Colleges and their associated bodies have identified audit departments. Department names and contact addresses are shown where appropriate. Some of the Colleges receive core clinical audit funding.

Royal College of Anaesthetists

Professional Standards Committee
Royal College of Anaesthetists
48–49 Russell Square
London WC1B 4JY

Tel: 020 7813 1900; fax: 020 7813 1876
URL: www.rcoa.ac.uk/menu6.html

Produces and disseminates guidelines for both clinical practice and audit methodology. Recently published *Raising the Standards*, a compendium of audit recipes.

Royal College of General Practitioners (RCGP)

Clinical and Special Projects Network
14 Princes Gate
Hyde Park
London SW7 1PU

Tel: 020 7581 3232; fax: 020 7225 3047
URL: www.rcgp.org.uk/rcgp/clinspec/index.asp

A newly created unit, St. Paul RCGP Quality Unit has been formed as part of the network to help raise standards in general practice. It will support individuals and organisations that are looking for a clear way to improve good clinical practice and quality of care.

The Royal College of General Practice also has an Effective Clinical Practice Unit at the University of Sheffield, which develops guidelines and includes the Clinical Practice Evaluation Unit.

Effective Clinical Practice Unit
University of Sheffield
Regent Court
30 Regent House
Sheffield S1 4DA

Tel: 0114 2220811

Royal College of Obstetricians & Gynaecologists

Audit Unit
27 Sussex Place
London NW1 4RG

Tel: 020 7772 6200
Fax: 020 7772 6390
URL: www.rcog.org.uk

The audit unit of this College coordinates national audits including the national sentinel audit of Caesarean section.

Royal College of Ophthalmologists

Audit Department
17 Cornwall Terrace
London NW1 4QW
URL: www.rcophth.ac.uk/

Tel: 020 7935 0702
e-mail: rco.audit@btinternet.com

The audit unit conducts both major audit projects and supports local audit. It can provide advice on planning audits, setting standards and determining outcomes.

Royal College of Paediatrics and Child Health

Research Division
Royal College of Paediatrics and Child Health
50 Hallam Street
London W1N 6DR

Tel: 020 7307 5674
Fax: 020 7307 5690
URL: www.rcpch.ac.uk

Within the research unit, a Clinical Effectiveness Coordinator maintains comprehensive databases of clinical audit projects and clinical guidelines. The Royal College of Paediatrics and Child Health coordinates national audits and is active in clinical guideline development in specific fields. It has produced an extremely useful guide to Internet sites.

Royal College of Pathologists

Clinical Audit and Effectiveness
2 Carlton House Terrace
London SW1Y 5AF

Tel: 020 7451 6732
Fax: 020 7451 6702
e-mail: audit@rcpath.org
URL: www.rcpath.org/activities/audit.html

This department aims to offer support for clinical audit activities for anyone wishing to undertake clinical audit in pathology. It maintains a database of clinical audits in a variety of specialties in pathology.

Royal College of Physicians

Clinical Effectiveness and
  Evaluation Unit
11 St. Andrew's Place
London NW1 4LE

Tel: 020 7935 1174
Fax: 020 7487 3988
e-mail: CEEU@rcplondon.ac.uk
URL: www.rcplondon.ac.uk/college.ceeu_home.htm

This unit produces clinical guidelines, designs audit tools, coordinates audit projects and develops clinical outcome measures.

Royal College of Psychiatrists

College Research Unit
17 Belgrave Square
London SW1X 8PG

Tel: 020 7235 2351 ext 234
Fax: 020 76245 1231
URL: www.rcpsych.ac.uk/cru

The College Research Unit is a department of this Royal College that emphasises 'getting research into practice' by producing clinical practice guidelines and organising national clinical audit projects amongst its other activities.

Royal College of Radiologists

Clinical Audit Advisor
38 Portland Place
London W1N 4JQ

Tel: 020 7636 4432
Fax: 020 7323 3100
e-mail: enquiries@rcr.ac.uk
URL: www.rcr.ac.uk

This college sets standards for members' participation in audit activity, disseminates guidelines and issues a guide for others to make the best use of a department of radiology.

Royal College of Surgeons of England

Clinical Effectiveness Unit
Royal College of Surgeons
   of England
35–43 Lincoln's Inn Fields
London WC2A 3PN

Tel: 020 7869 6600
Fax: 020 7869 6644
URL: www.rcseng.ac.uk/public/ceu/default.asp

This unit supports both national and comparative audits and research.

Journals and/or periodicals

The following are a list of publications with a primarily clinical governance and/or audit emphasis. There are many other publications concentrating on general healthcare quality matters that are not included here.

British Journal of Clinical Governance

MCB University Press
60/62 Toller Lane
Bradford
West Yorkshire BD8 9BY

Tel: 01274 777 700
Fax: 01274 785 200
URL: www.mcb.co.uk

Quarterly; subscription (2000): UK £150 + VAT.

Clinical Governance Bulletin

RSM Press
1 Wimpole Street
London W1G 0AE

Tel: 020 7290 2923
Fax: 020 7290 2929
URL: www.clinical-governance.com

Bimonthly; Individual annual subscription: £30 (Europe), $54 (USA), £32 (rest of world); Institutional annual subscription: £50 (Europe), $90 (USA), £52 (rest of world).

Journal of Clinical Governance

Department of General Practice
University of Leicester
Leicester General Hospital
Gwendolen Road
Leicester LE5 4PM

Tel: 0116 258 4873

Quarterly; subscription (2000): UK £50; Overseas £55.

Network

Newsletter of the Clinical Audit Association
Clinical Audit Association Ltd.
Cleethorpes Business Centre
Jackson Place
Wilton Road
Humberston
North East Lincolnshire DN36 4AS

Tel/fax: 01472 210 682

Bimonthly; subscription (2000): £25; free to members of the Clinical Audit Association.

Healthcare Quality

Journal of the Association for Quality in Healthcare   **Tel:** 0118 981 6666
Association for Quality in Healthcare   **Fax:** 0118 981 9801
Portland House
Aldermaston Park
Reading
Berks RG7 4HR
Bimonthly; subscription (annual) £65; free to members of the Association for Quality in Healthcare.

Quality in Healthcare

BMJ Publishing Group   **Tel:** 020 7383 6270
PO Box 299   **Fax:** 020 7383 6402
London WC1H 9TD   **e-mail:** Subscriptions@bmjgroup.com
                        URL: www.qualityhealthcare.com
Quarterly; subscriptions (2000): £130 institutional; £80 individual.

Confidential enquiries:

The four Confidential Enquiries now come under the aegis of the NICE. Participation in the National Confidential Enquiry into Perioperative Deaths (NCEPOD) is now compulsory.

Confidential Enquiry Into Suicide & Homicide By People With Mental Illness

PO Box 86   **Tel:** 0161 291 4751/4752
Manchester M20 2EF   **Fax:** 0161 291 4358

Confidential Enquiries into Maternal Deaths (CEMD)

Room 520   **Tel:** 020 7972 4344;
Wellington House   **Fax:** 020 7972 4348
133–155 Waterloo Road
London SE1 8UG

Confidential Enquiries into Stillbirths & Deaths in Infancy (CESDI)

Chiltern Court   **Tel:** 020 7486 1191
188 Baker Street   **Fax:** 020 7486 6543
London NW1 5SD   **e-mail:** director@cesdi.org.uk
                        URL: www.cesdi.com

Confidential Enquiries into Counselling for Genetic Disorders

Genetic Enquiry Centre, 6th Floor   **Tel:** 0161 276 6262
St Mary's Hospital   **Fax:** 0161 248 8308
Manchester   **e-mail:** rodney.harris@man.ac.uk

National Confidential Enquiry into Peri-operative Deaths (NCEPOD)
35–43 Lincoln's Inn Fields   **Tel:** 020 7831 6430
London WC2A 3PN   **Fax:** 020 7430 2958
                            e-mail: info@ncepod.org.uk
                            URL: http://www.ncepod.org.uk

National audit activities:

Specialist groups, associations and bodies often coordinate national audits. The following is not an exhaustive list. Some of these studies are partially centrally funded. Participation in these audits is usually voluntary and sometimes a fee is required from the participant.

Audit Of Intensive Care And High Dependency Care
Intensive Care National Audit and Research Centre (ICNARC)
Tavistock House   **Tel:** 020 7388 2856
Tavistock Square   **Fax:** 020 7388 3759
London WC1H 9HR   **e-mail:** kathy@icnarc.demon.co.uk

National Comparative Audit
Royal College of Surgeons of England   **Tel:** 020 7869 6610
35–43 Lincoln's Inn Fields   **Fax:** 020 7831 9483
London WC2A 3PN

Nosocomial Infection National Surveillance Scheme (NINS)
Nosocomial Infection Surveillance Unit **Tel:** 020 8200 4400
Central Public Health Laboratory   **Fax:** 020 8205 9185
61 Colindale Avenue   **URL:** www.phls.co.uk
London NW9 5HT

UK Trauma Audit and Research Network
Clinical Sciences Building
University of Manchester   **Tel:** 0161 787 4397
Hope Hospital   **Fax:** 0161 787 4345
Salford   **e-mail:** dyates@fslho.man.ac.uk;
Manchester M6 8HD   maralynw@fslho.man.ac.uk
                          URL: www.hop.man.ac.uk/uktrauma

Courses:

Since clinical (originally medical) audit was first identified as a mandatory quality assurance activity in healthcare in 1989, a number of courses have been developed to enhance the professional development of those working in this field. Some of these courses now result in a recognised professional qualification. The following list is by no means exhaustive – new ones are being developed all the time.

National Certificate in Clinical Audit

This is a flexible learning programme established in 1998, aimed at enabling those who have been working in the field of clinical audit to gain a recognised qualification utilising their existing experience and work.

Patricia Kent
Clinical Audit Association Ltd.   **Tel/fax:** 01472 210 682
Cleethorpes Business Centre   **e-mail:** pmkent@the-caa-ltd.demon.co.uk
Jackson Place, Wilton Road
Humberston
North East Lincs DN36 4AS

Clinical Audit and Effectiveness

This is a modular course which results in either a certificate (after one year), a diploma (after two years) or an MSc (after three years following dissertation). The course aims to provide the knowledge, skills and understanding necessary for a healthcare professional to promote, support and/or undertake evidence-based clinical practice.

School of Postgraduate Studies in Medical
    and Healthcare   **Tel:** 01792 703 578
University of Wales   **Fax:** 01792 797 310
Morriston Hospital   **e-mail:** pmschool@swansea.ac.uk
Swansea SA6 6NL   **URL:** www.swansea.ac.uk/pmschool

MSc in Evaluation of Clinical Practice

This is a two-year part-time day-release course leading to an MSc degree.

University of Westminster   **Tel:** 020 7911 5883
115 New Cavendish Street   **Fax:** 020 7911 5079
London W1M 8JS   **e-mail:** cavadmin@wmin.ac.uk

Basic Audit Training

This is a three-day foundation course for those new to clinical audit.

PMK Training Associates   **Tel:** 01472 813 258
25 Westport Road, Cleethorpes   **Fax:** 01472 813 258
North Lincolnshire DN35 0QF

Please note PMK Training Associates also provide a number of courses to develop and enhance the skills required by audit professionals such as questionnaire design, interview techniques, statistics etc. Further details can be obtained from the address above.

Using Clinical Audit to Improve Clinical Effectiveness

A five-day course for those supporting clinical audit and clinical effectiveness programmes.

Healthcare Quality Quest   **Tel:** 01703 814 024
Shelley Farm   **Fax:** 01703 814 020
Shelley Lane, Ower
Romsey
Hants SO51 6AS

A range of courses is available relating to clinical audit, clinical governance and quality improvement. Consultancy service is also provided to independently review inhouse audit departments. Further details can be obtained from the address above.

Assessment of Health Needs

Assessment of health needs may be broken down into two elements:

▶ Healthcare needs assessment concentrates on healthcare services.

▶ Health needs assessment aims to assess the overall health of a defined community.

Healthcare needs assessment

Stevens and Raftery (1997; see below) define healthcare needs as 'the population's ability to benefit from healthcare'. Information is commonly collected in three ways:

Epidemiological needs assessment: Published and local information on the incidence and prevalence of a disease, together with evidence of interventions effectiveness, are used to define the needs of the local population (ie how many people could benefit by how much from a given service). This is the gold standard for evidence-based practice. Increasingly, the information needed to complete an epidemiological needs assessment will be available through NICE.

Comparative needs assessment: This compares services, activity and routine health data within and between districts to identify significant differences. When using this approach, it is difficult to distinguish between what is *needed* to improve health, what is *supplied* by local professional and what is *demanded* by local people. The three are not the same.

Corporate needs assessment: This takes account of the opinions and wishes of local people, GPs, providers, national and regional policy-makers and other agencies. Again, there may be a blurring of needs and demand.

Health needs assessment aims to assess the overall health of the community. The community may be defined geographically, culturally or administratively, such as a General Practice population. Commonly, a three-pronged approach is used.

▶ Collate routine data on births, morbidity, use of health and social care services, mortality and social indicators, such as unemployment, which affect health.

▶ Establish the community's own assessment of their health and health needs, through questionnaires, individual interviews or focus groups.

▶ Ascertain the views of key individuals and organisations as to the health and health needs of the community.

Sources of information on needs assessment methodology

Books:

Abramson JH. *Survey Methods in Community Medicine*, 5th Edition. London: Harcourt Publishers Ltd, 1998.
Annett H, Rifkin SB. *Guidelines for Rapid Participatory Appraisal to Assess Community Health Needs: a Focus for Health Improvements for Low-Income Urban and Rural Areas.* Geneva: WHO, 1995.

Gillam SJ, Murray SA. *Needs Assessment in General Practice*. Occasional Paper 73. London: Royal College of General Practitioners, 1996.

Harris A (ed). *Needs to Know: A Guide to Needs Assessment for Primary Care*. London: Royal Society of Medicine Press, 1997.

Hawtin M. *Community Profiling: Auditing Social Needs*. Buckingham: Open University Press, 1994.

Last JM. *A Dictionary of Epidemiology*, 3rd Edition. Oxford: Oxford University Press, 1995.

Robinson J, Elkan R. *Health Needs Assessment: Theory and Practice*. Edinburgh: Churchill Livingstone, 1996.

Sanderson HG, Mountney LM, Anthony PA. *Casemix for All*. Oxford: Radcliffe Medical Press, 1998.

Stevens A, Raftery J. *Healthcare Needs Assessment – the Epidemiologically Based Needs Assessment Reviews*, 2nd series. The Wessex Institute. Radcliffe Medical Press, 1997.

Wright J. Health *Needs Assessment in Practice*. London: BMJ Publishing Group, 1998.

Papers:

Gillam S. Assessing the health needs of populations – the general practitioners contribution. *British Journal of General Practice* 1992; 42: 404–405.

Jordan J, Dowswell T, Harrison S, Lilford R. Whose priority? Listening to users and the public. *British Medical Journal* 1998; 316: 1668–1670.

Jordan J, Wright J. Making sense of health needs assessment at a practice level; using routine data in a meaningful way. *Journal of Public Health* 1998; 19(3): 255–261.

Murray S, Graham L. Practice based health needs assessment: use of four methods in a small neighbourhood. *British Medical Journal* 1995; 310: 1443–1448.

Ruta DA, Duffy MC, Farquharson A. Determining priorities for change in primary care: the value of practice based needs assessment. *British Journal of General Practice* 1997; 47: 353–357.

Shanks J, Kheraj S, Fish S. Better ways of assessing health needs in primary care. *British Medical Journal* 1995; 308: 480–481.

Slade M. Thornicroft G. User-friendly assessment of need. *Nursing Times* 1999; 95(33): 52–53, Aug 18-24.

Stevens A, Gabbay J. Needs assessment needs assessment…. *Health Trends* 1991; 23(1): 20–21.

Stevens A, Gillam S. Needs assessment from theory to practice. *British Medical Journal* 1998; 316: 1448–1452.

Wilkinson M. Assessment in primary care: practical issues and possible approaches. *British Medical Journal* 1998; 316: 1524–1528.

Williams R, Wright J. Epidemiological issues in health needs assessment. *British Medical Journal* 1998; 316: 1379–1382.

Wright J, William R, Wilkinson J. Development and importance of health needs assessment. *British Medical Journal* 1998; 316: 1310–1313.

NHS IMG Reference G7108. *A Methodology for the Health Benefit Group Development Project.* Available from the National Casemix Office, Information Management Group, NHS Executive Headquarters, Highcroft, Romsey Road, Winchester S022 5DH. Tel: 01962 844 588.

Organisations:

Faculty of Public Health
4 St. Andrews Place
London NW1 4LB
Tel: 020 7935 0243

Public Health Forum
Contributions to:
John Fox
Office for National Statistics
1 Drummond Gate
London SW1V 2QQ
Distribution:
Katie Stone
King's Fund
11–13 Cavendish Square
London W1M 0AN

Royal College of Nursing
20 Cavendish Square
London W1M 9AE
Tel: 020 7409 3333

Association of Public Health
Trevelyan House
30 Great Peter Street
London SW1P 0HW
Tel: 020 7413 1896

Websites:

Faculty of Public Health Medicine
http://www.fphm.org.uk/fphm.htm

First Report of the National Screening Committee
This contains the criteria by which a screening test should be assessed.
http://www.doh.gov.uk/nsc/pdfs/nsc_firstreport.pdf

Examples of Good Practice Involving Patients
http://www.open.gov.uk/doh/pcharter/phctip3.htm

Undertaking Systematic Reviews of Research on Effectiveness
NHS Centre for Reviews and Dissemination (CRD) guidelines for those carrying out or commissioning reviews.
CRD report number 4 January 1996.
http://www.york.ac.uk/inst/crd/report4.htm

Health Needs Assessment in Primary Healthcare: A Workbook for Primary Healthcare Teams (Version 2) – September 1998
Dr Judith Hooper   **URL:** www.geocities.com/HotSprings/4202/hnawrk.html
Phil Longworth
Calderdale and Kirklees Health Authority
Huddersfield

Courses:

Most universities run MSc courses in Public Health. Often, these are modular, allowing an individual to tailor the course of their own needs. The most well-known courses is at the London School of Hygiene and Tropical Medicine
Keppel Street
London WC1E 7HT
Course organiser: Dr Aileen Clarke. Tel: 020 7636 8636.

Clinical Risk Management

Clinical risk management is a mechanism for managing exposure to risk that enables us to recognise the damaging consequences in the future, their severity and how they can be controlled.

Dickson G. Principles of risk management. *Quality in Healthcare* 1995; 4: 75–79.

Organisations:

ALARM (Association of Litigation and Risk Management)
Objectives / Activities:

▶ To improve patient care by promoting effective risk management.

▶ To cut the cost of litigation by encouraging best practice in the investigation and management of claims.

▶ To provide a forum for risk and claims managers to share experiences, exchange information and develop solutions to clinical risk and claims management problems.

Membership is corporate, and named representatives are responsible for managing clinical negligence claims and the implementation of clinical risk management programmes.

Three seminars per year are held in London and a newsletter is produced for members. There are also regular training courses in relevant topics.

Contact: Margaret Dangoor
Executive Director
ALARM
3 Clydesdale Gardens
Richmond
Surrey TW10 5EG
Tel: 020 8241 3815

Chesterfield Clinical Risk Management Group
Contact: Brian Gibbs
Director of Support Services
Bassetlaw Hospital and Community Services NHS Trust
Bassetlaw District General Hospital
Kilton
Worksop S81 0BD
Tel: 01909 500 990; fax: 01909 502 810

CNST (Clinical Negligence Scheme for Trusts)
Objectives / activities:

▶ To set and auditing of clinical risk management standards for member Trusts.

▶ To issue the periodical newsletter and guidance.

▶ To hold roadshows to raise awareness and knowledge.

Contact: Roger Mason
Risk Management Co-ordinator
Howard House
Queens Avenue
Bristol BS8 1SN
Tel: 0117 926 2091; fax: 0117 929 9845

Assessors: Sarah Hepworth (North of England)   0191 253 5723
Wendy Huxley Marko (Midlands)   0156 879 7667
Caroline Brown (South of England)   0196 285 6940
Dominique Wright (Midlands)   01905 796 887
Moya Berry (South of England)   01483 306 983

Clinical Risk Unit (CRU)

The CRU was established in April 1995 with funding from the North Thames Health Agencies to continue and develop the North-West Thames risk management project. The CRU has focused on two main functions: (i) to design and run the North Thames training programme in risk management; and (ii) to carry out research into the cause and consequences of injury to patients, complaints and litigation and to develop effective methods of prevention.

For information on research contact:

Charles Vincent
Director of the Clinical Risk Unit   **Tel:** 020 7504 5948
Psychology Dept   **Fax:** 020 7391 1647
Clinical Risk Unit   **e-mail:** c.vincent@ucl.ac.uk
1–19 Torrington Place
University College London
Gower Street
London WC1E 6BT
See Training section for contacts for CRU courses.

Health Services Management Centre (HSMC)

The HSMC undertakes health service research. Kieran Walshe and Maria Dineen have a particular interest in research in clinical risk management, claims, clinical effectiveness and clinical governance.

Contact: Maria Dineen
Health Service Management Centre
Park House
40 Edgbaston Road   **Tel:** 0121 414 7050
Birmingham B15 2RT   **Pager:** 01523 523 523 Code: 658604

Litigation and Risk Management Network

Objectives / activities:

This network comprises claims managers, risk managers, legal service managers, health and safety managers and others with similar responsibilities for all types of Trusts and Health Authorities from Northern Yorkshire and Yorkshire and Trent Regions.

Those involved meet quarterly at Pinderfields Hospital, Wakefield, to network, share problems and experiences, keep up to date with current topics, benchmark activities / procedures, hear guest speakers, and so on.

Contact: Michael O'Connell
Legal Services Manager
Pinderfields Hospitals NHS Trust **Tel:** 0192 421 3842
Trust HQ **Fax:** 0192 481 4929
Rowan House
Pinderfields General Hospital
Aberford Road
Wakefield WF1 4EE

London Clinical Risk Forum

Objectives / activities:

Informal gathering, open to any risk managers based in central London who have a remit for clinical risk management. The principle objective is to share best practice and experiences openly.

Contact: Finola Devaney
Assistant Clinical Risk Manager
Great Ormond Street Hospital **Tel:** 020 7813 8185
Great Ormond Street
London WC1N 3JH

Medical Defence Union (MDU)

Clinical Risk Department **Tel:** 0161 428 1234
192 Altrincham Road
Sharston
Manchester M22 4RZ

Northern Risk Management Forum

Objectives / activities:

- To be a forum for networking with colleagues involved in the field of risk management.

- To invite guest speakers on topics of interest to the forum.

- To share experiences in the field of risk management.

- To hold site visits and benchmarking opportunities.

Contact: Henry Stahr
Centre for Advanced Inter-Professional Development
Continuing Education Unit
The University of Salford
Salford M5 4WT

Royal College of Anaesthetics

Catherine Arden, Director, Professional Standards Directorate
Royal College of Anaesthetics   **Tel:** 020 7813 1900
48–49 Russell Square   **URL:** www.rcoa.ac.uk
London WC1B 4JY

Information on the College's pilot study and database for anaesthetic critical incident reporting can be accessed via the College's website.

STORM (Scottish Trust Officers in Risk Management)

Objectives / activities:

This is an informal network of about 40 people, meeting occasionally to discuss matters of mutual interest.

Contact: Dr Terence Nunn
Associate Hospital Medical Director
Law Hospital NHS Trust   **Tel:** 01698 361 100
Carluke   **Fax:** 01698 376 671
Lanarkshire ML8 5ER

Welsh Risk Pool

Objectives / activities:

▶ Administration of self-insurance pool for Wales, including clinical negligence and personal injury.

▶ To hold occasional courses / seminars on risk management.

Contact: Ian Biggs, Manager
HM Stanley Hospital   **Tel:** 01745 589 743
St. Asaph
Denbyshire WL17 0RS

West Midlands Clinical Consortium

Contact: Maria Dineen
Health Services Management Centre
Park House   **Tel:** 0121 414 7050
40 Edgbaston Road   **Pager:** 01523 523 523 Code 658604
Birmingham B15 2RT

Yorkshire Clinical Risk Co-ordinators Group

Objectives / activities:

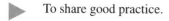 To share good practice.

- To provide a 'hands on', problem-solving approach for issues raised by members of the group.

- Information exchange between members.

- To ensure peer support for clinical risk coordinators.

- To facilitate standard-setting for clinical risk issues within the membership of the group.

- To provide a focal point for all clinical risk issues.

- To identify training needs and stimulate or provide training and continued education.

The group meets bimonthly, with additional special interest groups as and when appropriate.

Contact: Julie Finch
        Clinical Risk Coordinator
        Bradford Hospitals NHS Trust   **Tel:** 01274 364 648
        Bradford Royal Infirmary
        Duckworth Lane
        Bradford BD9 6RJ

Journals / books:

Clinical Risk Management
Editor: Charles Vincent
Published by the BMJ Publishing Group, 1995

Medical Negligence and Clinical Risk: Trends and Developments
Vivienne Harpwood
Published by Monitor Press Ltd., 1998
Suffolk House
Church Field Road
Sudbury
Suffolk CO10 6YA

Risk Management in the NHS
NHS Management Executive
Leeds: NHSME, 1993

Clinical Risk
Publications subscriptions department
Royal Society of   **Tel:** 020 7290 2928
   Medicine Press Ltd.   **Fax:** 020 7290 2929
1 Wimpole Street   **e-mail:** rsmjournals@rsm.ac.uk
London W1G 0AE   **URL:** www.rsmpress.ac.uk; www.rsm.ac.uk/pub/cr.htm
Bimonthly; subscription (annual): £142 (Europe), $253 (USA), £146 (elsewhere).

Healthcare Risk Report

The Marketing department   **Tel:** 020 7354 5858
The Eclipse Group   **Fax:** 020 7354 8106
18–20 Highbury Place
London N5 1QP
Published ten times a year; subscription: £260 per annum.

Health Law for Healthcare Professionals

This is a concise and informative review of the latest legal, financial and administrative developments that dictate how organisations care for patients.
Monitor Press Ltd.   **Tel:** 01787 467 223
Suffolk House   **Fax:** 01787 881 147
Church Field Road
Sudbury
Suffolk CO10 6YA
Ten issues per year; subscription: £172 per annum.

Medical Law Monitor

Monthly medico-legal newsletter summarising the most pertinent and influential cases likely to affect strategic and operational decision-making.
Monitor Press Ltd.   **Tel:** 01787 467 223
Suffolk House   **Fax:** 01787 881 147
Church Field Road
Sudbury
Suffolk CO10 6YA
Monthly; subscription: £226 per annum.

Managing Medical Risk

Thames Media International Ltd.   **Tel:** 020 8699 2220
7 Courtrai Road   **Fax:** 020 8699 3735
London SE23 1PL
Quarterly; subscription: £25 per annum

Courses:

Centre for Health Informatics and Multiprofessional Education (CHIME at UCL)

Since January 1999, University College London formalised the training conferences on clinical risk management that had been running with the Clinical Risk Unit and at North Thames Region, to create three postgraduate part-time programmes. The risk management qualifications are:

- MSc: Eight taught modules + a dissertation (2 years)

- Diploma: Eight taught modules (1.5–2 years)

- Certificate: Four taught modules (1 year)

Courses are two days teaching a month at UCL plus ten hours home study per week. The primary focus is on clinical risk management, examining what goes wrong in medicine and patient care and how to minimise risks. Psychological, legal and financial issues are addressed. Organisational factors and systems analyses are examined as a method of reducing blame culture. The course has a strong research basis and training is given in critical appraisal of literature and in running research projects. Topics include:

- Risk management principles

- Organisational risk

- Medical law

- Research design and statistics

- Selection, training and monitoring of performance

- Psychological responses to stress and trauma

- Health and safety

- Art and science of communication

- Access to information

- Finance.

The course is aimed at senior health service staff. At present, our 27 students include consultant and SpR doctors, directors of nursing/quality, senior nurses and risk managers. The minimum requirements are a second class degree in a health-related subject, law or psychology, plus five years in the health sector. Applicants without a degree can enrol on the diploma and upgrade to the MSc.

For further information, contact Pippa Bark at:

Royal Free and University College Medical School

CHIME, Archway Campus **Tel:** 020 7288 3383

Highgate Hill **Fax:** 020 7288 3389

London N19 3UA **e-mail:** p.bark@chime.ucl.ac.uk

URL: www.chime.ucl.ac.uk/MedEd/Courses/MScRM/

Clinical Effectiveness

Clinical effectiveness encompasses the concept that healthcare treatments should be effective and cost-effective, and that evidence on the efficacy of treatments should be sought from well-conducted research. It involves assessing the research evidence to determine whether interventions work, presenting the findings on what is most effective, and disseminating those findings to encourage changes in practice. Information on the clinical effectiveness of interventions should ideally come from well-conducted systematic reviews of primary studies, and may be disseminated in a variety of formats.

The following list of key organisations, programmes and information resources is necessarily selective and is biased towards the UK.

Organisations:

Aggressive Research Intelligence Facility (ARIF)

This is an initiative funded by the West Midlands Regional Office to provide support to purchasers in finding and interpreting research evidence to inform decisions. The summaries of ARIF's findings on specific effectiveness questions are available on the Internet.

Department of Public Health and Epidemiology

University of Birmingham	**Tel/fax:** 0121 414 7878
Edgbaston	**e-mail:** c.j.hyde@bham.ac.uk
Birmingham B15 2TT	**URL:** www.hsrc.org.uk/links/arif/arifhome.htm

Cochrane Collaboration

This comprises a worldwide network of researchers producing methodologically rigorous systematic reviews of the effectiveness of healthcare interventions based primarily on assessments of the evidence from randomised controlled trials. The reviews are published as the Cochrane Database of Systematic Reviews, which is available as part of the Cochrane Library (a collection of databases available on CD-ROM and via the World Wide Web). The Collaboration also compiles the Cochrane Controlled Trials Register: a unique collection of more than 260 000 controlled clinical trials (the raw material for many systematic reviews).

Information on the Cochrane Collaboration can be obtained from:

UK Cochrane Centre	**Tel:** 01865 516 300
Summertown Pavilion	**Fax:** 01865 516 311
Middle Way	**e-mail:** general@cochrane.co.uk
Oxford OX2 7LG	**URL:** www.imbi.uni-freiburg.de/cochrane

Information on the Cochrane Library can be obtained from:

Update Software	**Tel:** 01865 513 902
Summertown Pavilion	**Fax:** 01865 516 918
Middle Way	**e-mail:** update@cochrane.co.uk
PO Box 696	**URL:** www.update-software.com/ccweb/
Oxford OX2 7LG	cochrane/cdsr.htm

Health Evidence Bulletins – Wales

These bulletins summarise the research evidence on key questions across broad categories of healthcare, such as maternal and early child health. The sources of evidence are clearly referenced and reports are available in full on the Internet.

Duthie Library	**Tel:** 029 2074 5142
University of Wales College	**Fax:** 029 2074 3651
of Medicine	**e-mail:** weightmanal@cardiff.ac.uk
Cardiff CF4 4XN	**URL:** www.uwcm.ac.uk/uwcm/lb/pep/index.html

NHS Centre for Reviews and Dissemination (CRD)

This is funded by the UK Departments of Health to provide information on the effectiveness and cost-effectiveness of healthcare interventions and ways of organising healthcare. CRD carries out systematic reviews and publishes evidence-based summaries and patient leaflets. CRD's reviews frequently use evidence from study designs other than randomised controlled trials. CRD promotes access to other sources of clinical effectiveness information by producing databases and providing training in how to find research evidence. The main products of CRD are set out below:

- Effective healthcare bulletins – summaries of the research evidence on the effectiveness of interventions, designed for decision-makers.

- Effectiveness matters – brief bulletins on key messages from research.

- Database of Reviews of Abstracts of Effectiveness (DARE) – critical summaries of quality assessed systematic reviews.

- NHS Economic Evaluation Database – critical summaries of economic evaluations of healthcare interventions.

- Health Technology Assessment database – author abstracts of technology assessment reports and ongoing projects undertaken by agencies around the world.

- Patient and practitioner leaflets – based on research evidence.

NHS Centre for Reviews and Dissemination (CRD)

University of York	**Tel:** 01904 433 707
York Y01 5DD	**Fax:** 01904 433 661
	e-mail: revdis@york.ac.uk
	URL: www.york.ac.uk/inst/crd

NHS Health Technology Assessment Programme

This programme prioritises and commissions research of importance to the NHS, which may include systematic reviews as well as primary research. The research results are published as Technology Assessment Reports and are available in print and on the Internet.

National Coordinating Centre for Health Technology Assessment
Mailpoint 728   **Tel:** 023 8059 5686
Boldrewood   **Fax:** 023 8059 5639
University of Southampton   **e-mail:** hta@soton.ac.uk
Southampton SO16 7PX   **URL:** www.hta.nhsweb.nhs.uk/main.htm

NICE

NICE is a Special Health Authority tasked with providing 'authoritative, robust and reliable guidance on current "best practice"'. Completed appraisals are provided on its website.

NICE   **Tel:** 020 7849 3444
90 Long Acre   **Fax:** 020 7849 3127
Covent Garden   **URL:** www.nice.org.uk/nice-web/
London WC2E 9RZ

Scottish Health Purchasing Information Centre (SHPIC)

This was a Scottish initiative to carry out and commission systematic reviews to inform health purchasing decisions in Scotland. Its reports are still available on the Internet.

A Scottish Health Technology Assessment Unit is now being established.
URL: www.nhsconfed.net/shpic/

Scottish Intercollegiate Guidelines Network (SIGN)

This network compiles evidence-based guidelines.

SIGN Secretariat
Royal College of Physicians   **Tel:** 0131 225 7324
   of Edinburgh   **Fax:** 0131 225 1769
9 Queen Street   **e-mail:** r.harbour@rcpe.ac.uk
Edinburgh EH2 1JQ   **URL:** www.show.scot.nhs.uk/sign/home.htm

Agency for Healthcare Research and Quality (AHRQ)

This US agency (formerly the Agency for Healthcare Policy and Research) conducted a series of large-scale reviews in the mid-1990s, which are available fulltext on the Internet. They are now producing evidence reports from evidence-based practice centres 'based on rigorous comprehensive syntheses and analyses of relevant scientific literature'.

Executive Office Center, Suite 600
2101 East Jefferson Street
Rockville   **e-mail:** info@ahrq.gov/
MD 20852   **URLs:** text.nlm.nih.gov/; www.ahcpr.gov/
USA

Canadian Task Force on Preventive Healthcare

Reviews of effective preventive care.
URL: www.ctfphc.org/; **e-mail**: ctf@ctfphc.org

US Preventive Services Task Force

Produce guidelines supplying research-based evidence on the effectiveness of preventive health strategies. Searchable by selecting 'Guide to Clinical Preventive Services. 2nd edition' from the Health Services/Technology Assessment Text (HSTAT) website search engine.

URL: text.nlm.nih.gov/

Databases:

Best Evidence

This is a CD-ROM product containing the fulltext of two journals: ACP Journal Club and Evidence-Based Medicine. These journals offer critical summaries of published research.

BMJ Publishing Group   **Tel:** 020 7387 4499
BMA House   **Fax:** 020 7383 6662
Tavistock Square   **URL:** www.acponline.org/catalog/journals/ebm.htm
London WC1H 9JR

Cochrane Database of Systematic Reviews

See Organisations: Cochrane Collaboration.

Cochrane Library

See Organisations: Cochrane Collaboration.

Database of Abstracts of Reviews of Effectiveness

See Organisations: NHS Centre for Reviews and Dissemination.

Evidence-Based Medicine Reviews (EBMR)

This is a recently launched database combining and linking the Cochrane Database of Systematic Reviews and Best Evidence to MEDLINE.

URL: www.ovid.com/index.cfm

NHS Economic Evaluation Database

See Organisations: NHS Centre for Reviews and Dissemination.

Journals and collections of effectiveness reports:

ACP Journal Club

This journal offers critical appraisals of primary research (such as randomised controlled trials and economic evaluations) and systematic reviews with a commentary from a clinical expert. The journal also is available as part of Best *Evidence* (see Databases).

URL: www.acponline.org/journals/acpjc/jcmenu.htm

Bandolier

This journal contains articles about the clinical effectiveness of interventions and ways of interpreting the research evidence. Available in print and fulltext on the Internet.

Hayward Medical Communications **Tel:** 01865 226 132
Rosemary House **Fax:** 01865 226 978
Lanwades Park **URL's:** www.ebando.com.uk/;
Kentford www.jr2.ox.ac.uk/bandolier
Near Newmarket
Suffolk CB8 7PW

Clinical Evidence

This is a compendium of evidence-based summaries of effectiveness, aimed primarily at primary care professionals.

BMJ Publishing **Tel:** 020 7387 4499
BMA House **Fax:** 020 7383 6662
Tavistock Square **URL:** www.evidence.org/
London WC1H 9JR

Drug and Therapeutics Bulletin

This journal reviews drugs and is aimed at UK GPs and pharmacists. It is available in print and on the British National Formulary CD-ROM.

DTB Department
Consumers' Association **Tel:** 01992 822 800
Castlemead **e-mail:** dtb@which.net
Gascoyne Way **URL:** www.which.net/health/dtb/main.html
Hertford SG14 1LH

Effective Healthcare Bulletins

See Organisations: NHS Centre for Reviews and Dissemination.

Effectiveness Matters

See Organisations: NHS Centre for Reviews and Dissemination.

Evidence-Based Medicine

This comprises critical appraisals of primary research (such as randomised controlled trials and economic evaluations) and systematic reviews, with a commentary from a clinical expert. The journal is also available on Best Evidence (see Databases).

BMJ Publishing Group **Tel:** 020 7387 4499
BMA House **Fax:** 020 7383 6662
Tavistock Square **URL:** www.bmjpg.com/data/ebm.htm/
London WC1H 9JR

British Journal of Clinical Governance (formerly Journal of Clinical Effectiveness)

This publishes papers on evidence-based practice, clinical effectiveness, guidelines and audit, and aims to be 'practical and clinically based'.

MCB University Press
60/62 Toller Lane
Bradford
West Yorkshire BD8 9BY

Tel: 01274 777 700
Fax: 01274 785 200
e-mail: liblink@liblink.co.uk
URL: www.mcb.co.uk/bjcg.htm

Indexes to clinical effectiveness resources:

Clinical effectiveness information is published in a variety of formats, many of which are not recorded by major databases, such as MEDLINE, which tend to concentrate on journal articles. The following Internet resources index many, but not all, of the key clinical effectiveness publications available on the WWW and offer searching by subject.

Turning Research Into Practice (TRIP)
This is the website of the TRIP initiative, part of CeReS (Centre for Research Support) in Gwent, Wales, maintained by Jon Brassey.
URL: www.ceres.uwcm.ac.uk/frameset.cfm?section=trip

ScHARR – Lock's Guide to the Evidence
Maintained by Andrew Booth of the School of Health and Related Research, University of Sheffield. It identifies material less likely to appear in the Cochrane Library or MEDLINE.
URL: www.shef.ac.uk/uni/academic/R-Z/scharr/ir/scebm.html

Guides to clinical effectiveness resources:

Netting the evidence: a ScHARR introduction to evidence based practice on the Internet.
http://www.shef.ac.uk/~scharr/ir/netting

NHS Executive Public Health Development Unit
Clinical effectiveness resource pack. London: Department of Health, 1997.
Available from NHS responseline, Tel: 0541 555 455 (catalogue number 97CC115) and fulltext at URL http://doh.gov.uk/pub/docs/doh/nhsfold.pdf

Implementation of clinical effectiveness information

Organisations and publications:

Evaluation of methods to promote the implementation of research findings
National programme of research coordinated by the London Regional Research and Development Directorate.
Melanie Baillie-Johnston
National R&D Commissioning Unit (North Thames)
R&D Directorate
40 Eastbourne Terrace
London W2 3QR
Tel: 020 7725 5395; fax: 020 7725 5467
e-mail: mjohnsop@doh.gov.uk; URL: www.doh.gov.uk/ntrd/rd/implem/index.htm

The Framework for Appropriate Care Throughout Sheffield (FACTS) Project

c/o ScHARR   **Tel:** 0114 275 5658
Regent Court   **Fax:** 0114 275 5653
30 Regent Street   **e-mail:** Facts@Sheffield.ac.uk
Sheffield S1 4DA   **URL:** www.shef.ac.uk/uni/projects/facts

ARIF

See Organisations: Aggressive Research Intelligence Function.

TRIP

See Indexes To Clinical Effectiveness Resources.

CHAIN (Contact Help Advice Information Network for Effective Healthcare)

This is a network, map and communication tool designed to facilitate links between professionals who are interested or active in evidence-based healthcare and clinical effectiveness.
URL: www.doh.gov.uk/ntrd/chain/chain.htm

Cochrane Effective Practice and Organisation of Care Review Group

This group reviews interventions designed to improve professional practice and the delivery of effective healthcare services. The group's reviews are published in the *Cochrane Library.*

Publications:

Dunning M, Abi-Aad G, Gilbert D, Hutton H, Brown C. *Experience, Evidence and Everyday Practice. Creating Systems for Delivering Effective Healthcare.* London: King's Fund, 1999.
This book reports on the findings of the PACE projects, and provides information on how to implement changes in clinical practice.

NHS Centre for Reviews and Dissemination. Getting evidence into practice. *Effective Healthcare*, 1999, 5(1).
Also available full text on the Internet at URL www.york.ac.uk/inst/crd/ehc51.htm

Palmer C, Fenner J. *Getting the Message Across.* London: Royal College of Psychiatrists, 1999.

Integrated Care Pathways

Integrated care pathways (ICPs):

> ... amalgamate all the anticipated elements of care and treatment of all members of the multidisciplinary team, for a patient or client of a particular case-type or grouping within an agreed time frame, for the achievement of agreed outcomes. Any deviation from the plan is documented as a 'variance'; the analysis of which provides information for the review of current practice.
>
> **Johnson S. Pathways of Care. Oxford: Blackwell Science, 1997**

or

> An ICP determines locally agreed, multidisciplinary practice based on guidelines and evidence where available, for a specific patient/client group. It forms part or all of the clinical record, documents the care given and facilitates the evaluation of outcomes for continuous quality improvement.
>
> **National Pathways Association, 1998**

There are many names for the pathway tool, which include the following:
Anticipated Recovery Pathways
Multidisciplinary Pathways of Care
CareMaps®
Critical Care Pathways
Care Profiles
Collaborative Care Pathways
Pathways of Care
Care Pathways

Organisations:

National Pathways Association (NPA)

This was formed in the early 1990s with local networks of pathway users around the UK. In 1994, the networks met together to form the National Pathway User Group (NPUG), which at the time provided a simple network for members. In October 1995, the NPUG became an official subscription-based organisation with a committee to administer the membership and the national quarterly meetings. In 1997, the NPUG changed its name to the National Pathways Association (NPA), to include non-pathway users into the membership. Membership now represents NHS Trusts from acute, community and mental health settings, primary care and private healthcare, plus Health Authorities and PCGs.

The NPA provides:

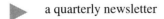 a quarterly newsletter

 a membership/contact list

 quarterly national meetings.

Carole Cairns (Fundraising and Publicity Board Member)
Priory Healthcare   **Tel:** 01895 836 339
Broadwater Park   **URL:** www.the-npa.org.uk
Denham
Uxbridge
Middlesex UB9 5HP

Scottish Pathway User Group

This group comprises a network of pathway users across Scotland. They host national meetings three times a year, and publish a newsletter. Membership is free. Recently, the focus of this group has moved towards the evaluation and review of pathways already in place.

It provides:

▶ a newsletter three times a year

▶ national meetings three times a year

▶ a database of contacts for all members.

Clinical Audit Office
West Glasgow Hospital
Glasgow G11 6NT

Journals, periodicals, books and reports:

The following gives an example of the many journals that now include articles on ICPs and related topics.

International Journal of Healthcare Quality Assurance
MCB University Press Ltd.   **Tel:** 01274 777700
60/62 Toller Lane   **Fax:** 01274 785200
Bradford
West Yorkshire BD8 9BY

Journal of Integrated Care Pathways (formerly Journal of Integrated Care)
Editor: Sue Johnson
Publishers: The Royal Society
    of Medicine Press   **Tel:** 020 7290 2927/8
PO Box 9002   **Fax:** 020 7290 2929
London W1A 0ZA   **e-mail:** rsmjournals@rsm.ac.uk
                               URL: www.rsmpress.ac.uk
Quarterly; subscriptions: £73 (Europe), $140 (US), £141 (rest of world)

NPA Newsletter
For members of the NPA.
See Organisations

Reports:

The Origins and Use of Care Pathways in the USA, Australia and the United Kingdom
Lynne Currie and Gill Harvey (1997)
Report No. 15, Royal College of Nursing
Dynamic Quality Improvement Programme
RCN Institute
Oxford Centre
Radcliffe Infirmary
Woodstock Road
Oxford OX2 6HE

Managing Care Pathways: The Quality And Resources Of Hospital Care
Authors: Jones de Luc and Coyne (1999), written for the ACCA
Publishers: ACCA
29 Lincoln's Inn Fields
London WC2A 3EE

Books:

Pathways of Care
Editor: Sue Johnson (1997)
Publishers: Blackwell Science
Osney Mead
Oxford OX2 0EL

Integrated Care Management; The Path To Success?
Editor: Jo Wilson (1997)
Publishers: Butterworth-Heinemann
Linacre House
Jordan Hill
Oxford OX2 8DP

Clinical Pathways Workbook
Sue Middleton and Adrian Roberts (1998)
Clinical Pathways Reference Centre   **Tel:** 01978 727 472
VFM Unit   **Fax:** 01978 727 470
Croesnewydd Hall
Wrexham Technology Park
Wrexham LL13 7YP
Wales

Integrated Care Pathways: A Practical Approach to Implementation
Authors: S Middleton and A Roberts
Publishers: Butterworth-Heinemann
Linacre House
Jordan Hill
Oxford OX2 8DP

Courses:

No courses exist that give a professional qualification; most ICP training exists as part of clinical audit, managed care or quality and management modules of professional training programmes. However, some independent parties do provide regular training on ICPs.

1) Venture Training and Consulting Ltd.
Directors: Sue Johnson and Jenny Gray
Chichester Office
40 Summerfield Road
West Wittering
Chichester
West Sussex PO20 8LY
Tel: 01243 514 463; fax: 01243 514 102
e-mail: info@venturetc.com; **URL:** www.venturetc.com

Specific courses provide:

- Introduction to ICPs (one day)
- How to write an ICP (one day)
- Variance tracking ICPs (one day)
- Managing an ICP project/programme (one day)
- ICP facilitator training course (three days)
- Facilitated workshops and many other tailored programmes
- Experienced consultancy support for ICP projects and developments.

2) Healthcare Risk Resources International Ltd.
Philip Nye
4th Floor, 40 Lime Street   **Tel:** 020 7220 7890
London EC3M 5EA   **Fax:** 020 7220 7891
                                             e-mail: pnye@hrri.co.uk
They provide tailored seminars on ICPs.

3) Kathryn de Luc and Sue Middleton
Chevington
Chevington Lane
Drakes Broughton
Worcester
Worcs WR10 2AE

Tel: 01386 553 311
e-mail: kathy@deluc.demon.co.uk

They provide basic training in the ICP tools, and how they are written.

4) Integrated Care Associates
Sue Middleton
19 Maxwell Close
Buckley
Flintshire CH7 3JE

Tel: 01244 545 042
Fax: 08700 527 646
e-mail: sue@suemiddleton-ica.demon.co.uk

They provide training in strategic planning for ICP projects/programmes and how to develop ICPs.

▶ Index

Note: page numbers in *italics* refer to figures and tables

Also available
from RSM Press

Medical Appraisal, Selection and Revalidation
A Professional's Guide to Good Practice
John Gatrell and Tony White

This book is a guide to appraising, recruiting and selecting consultants and junior doctors and focuses on the core skills required for making these decisions.

Based on extensive research involving over 600 medical interviews and numerous meetings with panel members and chairs, this book gives numerous examples of good practice and gathers together all available advice from a wide range of relevant sources including the NHS, BMA, Royal Colleges, GMC, deaneries, trusts and general practice. All the examples are taken from real interviews.

November 2000, 76pp, £12.95, ISBN: 1-85315-400-8

Medical Evidence
A Handbook for Doctors
Roger V. Clements, Roy Palmer, Neville Davis and Raina Patel

Doctors can appear in courts as defendants, witnesses and medical experts. This book is a guide to giving evidence in a range of different contexts including civil and criminal courts, coroner's courts, and occupational health and industrial tribunals. It explains clearly the relationship between the doctor and the law, highlighting the pitfalls of giving evidence, and examines the ethical and moral areas involved in individual cases. The New Civil Procedure Rules are explained in clear and simple terms.

April 2001, 106pp, £17.50, ISBN: 1-85315-387-7

Ordering information
Before 30 June 2001: Hoddle, Doyle, Meadows Ltd
Station Road, Linton, CAMBS CB1 6UX
Tel +44 (0)1223 893855   Fax +44 (0)1223 893852

After 30th June 2001: Marston Book Services
PO Box 269, Abingdon, Oxon OX14 4YN
Tel +44 (0)1235 465550   Fax +44 (0)1235 465555

Order online at www.rsmpress.co.uk

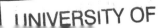